Today's Priorities in Mental Health

PRIORITY ISSUES IN MENTAL HEALTH

A book series published under the auspices of The World Federation for Mental Health

VOLUME 1

Today's Priorities in Mental Health

Children and Families - Needs, Rights, and Action

EDITORS

Stuart H. Fine, M.B.

Robert Krell, M.D.

Tsung-yi Lin, M.D.

ASSOCIATE EDITORS

Morton Beiser, M.D.

David S. Freeman, D.S.W.

Richard Nann, D.S.W.

CONTRIBUTING STAFF, WFMH

Roberta Beiser, Executive Director

Nora Curiston

Ann McCarthy

D. REIDEL PUBLISHING COMPANY

DORDRECHT : HOLLAND / BOSTON : U.S.A.

LONDON : ENGLAND

Library of Congress Cataloging in Publication Data

CIP

Main entry under title:

Today's priorities in mental health.

Papers presented at an international congress, held in Salzburg, Austria, co-sponsored by the Austrian Association for Mental Health and the World Federation for Mental Health.

Includes bibliographies and index.

1. Child mental health–Congresses. 2. Family–Mental Health–Congresses. I. Fine, Stuart H. II. Krell, Robert. III. Lin, Tsung-Yi. IV. World Federation for Mental Health. V. Austrian Association for Mental Health.

RJ499.T59 362.2'088054 80-23028

ISBN-13:978-94-009-9075-3 e-ISBN-13:978-94-009-9073-9
DOI: 10.1007/978-94-009-9073-9

Published by D. Reidel Publishing Company,
P.O. Box 17, 3300 AA Dordrecht, Holland.

Sold and distributed in the U.S.A. and Canada
by Kluwer Boston Inc.
190 Old Derby Street, Hingham, MA 02043, U.S.A.

In all other countries, sold and distributed
by Kluwer Academic Publishers Group,
P.O. Box 322, 3300 AH Dordrecht, Holland

D. Reidel Publishing Company is a member of the Kluwer Group

TABLE OF CONTENTS

SECTION FOUR – ISSUES WITH THERAPEUTIC IMPLICATIONS

SECTION FIVE – SPECIAL EVENTS

SECTION SIX – WORKSHOP REPORTS

PREFACE

Two themes seem to emerge repeatedly when reading through this volume. One is 'consensus' and the other is 'search'. There was a strong consensus during the Congress that children and families were the major and foremost concern of all present, regardless of their geographic origin or professional background. This concern was often expressed in terms of commitment to or as goal for the international mental health movement for the years to come.

The second theme, 'search', represents an effort to translate this concern into activities: search for concrete, immediate goals, for ways and means of translating into actual programs and projects, for interested people to carry on the work and better ways to train them to do the work well, for ways to obtain support, and lastly, search for ways of coordinating efforts of people in different parts of the world. All these and other matters are taken up in the discussions in this volume. The complexity of problems encountered in a rapidly changing world and the diversity of resources available in different parts of the world, make the task of searching difficult and sometimes confusing. In spite of the earnest efforts made, the results may be inconclusive and some of those proposed can be regarded only as hypotheses or ideas for experimentation. I trust this process of search will continue and the results of experimentation based on some of these hypotheses and theories will be fed back into the process of searching. This will help to make it more rewarding.

I should like to add another dimension to the process of search, that may or may not be apparent in the following chapters. This is the 'esprit de corps' of the participants who regard the Salzburg Congress as a second theatre of encounter and soul-searching, following the 1977 Vancouver Congress. 'Vancouver spirit' was characterized by shared concern for other human beings plus continuity of an endeavour by those who benefitted from the meeting and felt that they had been special to each other. This feeling would then be spread to others. Happily, this seems to have been well carried on to this Salzburg Congress.

Enhanced by the natural setting and rich cultural atmosphere of the historic city of Salzburg, the Vancouver spirit seems to have made another mark on the history of the World Federation for Mental Health in its effort to promote mental health to every corner of the world. The general theme of the Vancouver Congress, 'Today's Priorities in Mental Health: Knowing and Doing', is now being narrowed to a more specific one - 'Children and Families: Needs, Rights and Action'. The process from generality to specificity also represents the untiring efforts of the World Federation to come up with more specific, concrete and effective action programs relevant to different people living in different parts of the world. It is in this spirit that I recommend the following chapters of this volume to everyone who cares for mental health of oneself and one's fellow human beings.

The volume also reflects the great success of the Salzburg Congress, a success which would not have been possible without the untiring efforts and enormous support given by many people, in many capacities. We are sincerely indebted to all of these and wish we could list all of the names who deserve such recognition. However, we can mention only a few.

We give special thanks to our Austrian hosts: Dr. I. Leodolter, Austrian Minister of Health and Environmental Protection; Dr. W. Haslauer, Landeshauptmann of the Province of Salzburg; Mr. H. Salfenauer, Lord Mayor of the City of Salzburg; Prof. Dr. W. J. Revers, Rector of the University of Salzburg; Prof. Dr. H. Lechner, Director, Psychiatric-Neurological University Clinic Graz; Prof. Dr. P. Berner, Austrian Association for Mental Health; and Dr. A. Aranibar and Dr. R. Strobl who assisted Prof. Drs. Lechner and Berner. The Organizing Committee did a superb job of overall coordination of the Congress. This was achieved although many thousands of miles separated many of its members. The Austrian Association for Mental Health and the WFMH worked harmoniously as the joint sponsors. Subcommittees of this Organizing Committee were three. The Program Committee was chaired by Prof. Dr. H. Lechner and vice-chaired by Prof. Dr. P. Berner. Other key members were Dr. T. Y. Lin, Dr. M. Beiser, Dr. S. Fine, Dr. D. Freeman, Prof. Dr. G. Hofmann, Dr. R. Krell, Prof. Dr. K. Kryspin-Exner, Mrs. E. Morgan, Dr. R. Nann, Prof. Dr. E. Pakesch, Prof. Dr. E. Ringel, Prof. Dr. W. Spiel, Prof. Dr. H. Strotzka, Prof. Dr. W. Walcher, and Dr. M. Wagner. We were very fortunate in having assistance and cooperation from WHO and UNICEF whose input and support were invaluable. Also making a major contribution to the Congress Program were the Plenary Speakers and Chair people who provided daily inspirations. The Workshop Coordinators accepted the massive task of putting together sessions of high quality and interest. All who attended the Congress are particularly grateful to this group for providing an opportunity for stimulating involvement. Reports from these workshops will be published as a monograph series.

The Finance Committee was comprised of Mr. G. Guest, Treasurer WFMH, Vancouver, Canada and Dr. A. Aranibar, Graz, Austria.

Thirdly, the Secretarial Committee headed by Dr. A. Aranibar, Graz, Dr. R. Strobl, Vienna and Mrs. R. Beiser, Vancouver were immeasurably assisted by the efforts and great dedication of many staff and volunteers. In particular, Ms. A. H. McCarthy, Vancouver, Ms. Nora Curiston, Vancouver, and from Austria, Ms. Renate Scheinecker, Ms. Daniele Dohnal, Ms. Heidemarie Schwaiger and Ms. Brigitte Schwaiger, and the staff at the Kongresshaus, under the direction of Dr. Gerhard Gross.

Without the involvement of our loyal volunteers around the world, I can honestly say, the Congress would not have achieved the level of success it did.

Very special thanks to each of these special people. Our sincere appreciation is also extended to four organizations without whose financial support several of the workshops would not have had the privilege of involving top people in their specific areas. These were Grove School (USA), Laidlaw Foundation (Canada), the Leisure Development Center (Japan) and March of Dimes (USA).

And finally, the biggest 'thank you' goes to all of the participants at the Congress for their interest and efforts in the furthering of mental health the world over. Through this cooperative spirit, the Salzburg Congress became a reality, a success and a wonderfully active memory.

TSUNG-YI LIN, M. D.

SECTION ONE

DEVELOPMENTAL NEEDS

INTRODUCTION

It is appropriate to start this selection of papers with the Margaret Mead Memorial Lecture as a tribute to this remarkable scientist. The paper by Dr. Spock has many interesting and cogent observations that Dr. Mead would have enjoyed and appreciated.

In this section an attempt is made to look at the developmental needs of children in three different countries on three different continents. The authors discuss the needs of children and adolescents in very different ways. Mrs. Gachukia outlines a global approach, Dr. Lebovici describes the needs within a psychoanalytical conceptual framework, and Dr. Spock describes the developmental stages and his personal suggestions for intervention, particularly in regard to the education of children and of their teachers.

All the authors try to show how intervention may be most effective: Dr. Spock rues the inexperience of young doctors and their expectations that young mothers should pay good money and have to schedule appointments for advice – rather than obtaining advice when needed and at no cost; Dr. Lebovici emphasizes the baby's right to obtain care from the mother whatever her preconconceived notion of his temperament, sex, intelligence and appearance; and Mrs. Gachukia gives us some insight into the political and cultural climate in Kenya and how important it is to change the attitudes of some rural communities, for example in obtaining minimal nutritional standards for the babies. She and Spock emphasize the need for good day care and adequate learning.

Lebovici stresses the interplay of genetic, social and psychological factors but he ends by raising the question as to 'whether development can be ensured by satisfying social needs alone?'. Gachukia and Spock tacitly agree that all aspects of development need attention – the somatic, psychological and social – but the improvement in the lot of the child may require political action to change educational content and to change public attitudes.

STUART FINE, M.B.

S. H. Fine, R. Krell, and Tsung-yi Lin (Eds.), 'Today's Priorities in Mental Health' 3.

BENJAMIN M. SPOCK, M.D. (USA)

The First Margaret Mead Memorial Lecture

THE WIDER DIMENSIONS OF MENTAL HEALTH

I'm proud to be the first Margaret Mead lecturer. I was a friend of Margaret's and I was pediatrician for Catherine, her daughter. I had great admiration for her. She was extraordinarily perceptive and intuitive in her study of societies. She was courageous in popularizing anthropology. I don't know if you are aware of the beating she took from some of the academic anthropologists of her time, who, like some academicians in other fields, looked down on anyone who tried to educate the public and popularize the subject. She was indefatigable, always willing to take on more responsibilities, always ready to fight for a good cause.

What I want to do today, is to discuss three or four stages of development, not to expound on them, but to point out how our industrial societies fail to meet the needs of children and families. The United States, technically advanced, wealthy, highly educated, still has many of the same problems as a developing country, particularly our inadequate health care and education. It makes me want to jump up and shout to people from developing countries, "Don't follow us, unless you clearly realize what a mess we have made in many areas!"

In recent years fascinating studies have been made in the field of so called bonding, the attachment of the mother to her newborn baby. It's been discovered, and confirmed by studies in various countries, that if you allow a baby to be with the mother for 30 or 45 minutes right after birth – instead of being whisked off to a newborn nursery – this provides an amazing advantage for the mother's relationship to the baby and the baby's development from then on. Specifically, the mother will be more attentive to her baby at one month and at one year of age. She will, during physical examinations, want to stand nearer to her child than a mother who hasn't had this 30 or 45 minutes advantage. She will, much more often, look into her baby's eyes when speaking to it. Breast feeding will go on much longer, on the average. Her baby will have gained 1½ lb more weight by the age of 6 months. At 5 years, the child will have a higher IQ and a better vocabulary. Amazing that 30 minutes of contact right after birth can do that much! Obstetric departments, properly concerned with avoiding infection, have excluded the father and they have kept the baby away from the mother to give her rest. But it's horrifying to realize that in these respects, as in others, we have interfered with nature's pattern, in bringing about what we thought were improvements.

In medicine, as in so many other fields, we frequently lose sight of what our patients, our clients, really need, as we become preoccupied with our own technical interests. One of the reasons for the sad decline in breast feeding around

S. H. Fine, R. Krell, and Tsung-yi Lin (Eds.), 'Today's Priorities in Mental Health' 5–13.

the world was the fact that pediatricians were so pleased, back at the turn of the century, with their expertise in inventing their formulas.

Although I have never directly been a staff member of a child guidance clinic, I've been closely associated with guidance clinics in three of the teaching jobs that I had. Now, looking back, I recall that one clinic was obsessed with school phobias – any child brought to the door with a school phobia was immediately admitted despite a long waiting list. Another gave high priority to problems before the age of 5 years. Another one was fascinated with infantile autism. None of those three clinics would have admitted a mentally retarded child. They would explain to parents that other institutions were better equipped to take care of the diagnosis and the guidance of such cases, although that was not actually true at all; these child guidance clinics could have been of great help to retarded children and their parents.

There are other, more serious, faults that we health professionals can fall into. We can easily come to depersonalize our patients and, in the process, to depersonalize ourselves. We may elevate ourselves, at least slightly, above our clients. We can acquire pomposity without noticing it. I've been disconcerted, in reviewing the literature on bonding in the last few weeks, to see that those authors who are in the vanguard of trying to get rid of blind conventions are falling into such stuffy jargon as 'at risk' – a certain kind of baby is 'at risk'. They refer to a 'dyad' – this being simply the mother and the baby. Another expression is 'en face', meaning face to face; that's correct for French-speaking people, but that is rather pompous in the United States. I'm 76 years of age and I've never heard these phrases before. Better to stick to ordinary language. It's not only that we communicate better, but we remind ourselves that we are ordinary people too.

I want to discuss the second year of life, which is the first dramatic stage of independence. Independence around a year of age caused me a lot of trouble when I was first in pediatric practice. In groping for some training to help me answer mothers' questions I'd had, in addition to my pediatric training, a year's psychiatric residence. That didn't tell me anything except how to diagnose the manic depressive psychosis and schizophrenia. So I became involved in psychoanalytic training; but there was not much that seemed to help me answer mothers' questions either, at least at first. One of the problems that I was up against was finding how difficult 1-year-olds can be, at least for some parents. Feeding problems: babies who had eaten everything with relish and in a cooperative spirit up to one year, suddenly became choosey and adamant. They clamped their jaws shut and refused to take the things that the mother considered most healthful, like vegetables, eggs and milk.

Back in those days, a lot of ambitious parents started toilet training in the middle of the first year. If they had made any progress, this progress was apt to be shattered during the first half of the 2nd year when a baby suddenly realizes, "Hey! these are *my* bowels that are being co-opted by my mother." And the baby would refuse to cooperate.

Another problem was the frequency with which babies learn to say no. Not because they don't want to do something. In New York City, the favorite event of the day was being taken in the pram to Central Park. The mother would say, "Now do you want to get dressed and go to the park?" The baby would automatically say, "No!" Not because she didn't want to go to the park, but because she suddenly realized that she was an entity with desires and rights of her own. She wanted at least to be consulted before she was rushed into things. Some parents love this stage of development. They like to see spunkiness coming out. Others are absolutely shattered because they suddenly feel they have lost all control and the child is only 1½ years of age. What I'm leading up to is the need for counseling. What we have done in our industrial societies is destroy the natural counseling system that used to exist in the extended family. We have to substitute pediatricians and other kinds of counselors. One of the traditions that has grown up in pediatrics is that during the first 6 months the mother brings the baby once a month. During the last 6 months of the first year, every other month. In the 2nd year, every four months. After that, two times a year. Well, we carried on a child rearing study at Western Reserve University in which we wanted to track down some of the controversial problems of child rearing. It was a very sophisticated group of counselors. We started seeing parents for an hour every other week; and when the children were 10 years of age, we were *still* seeing the parents for an hour every other week. There was no dearth of things to talk about. I don't mean that in most cases there were serious problems, but that there were things that the mothers still needed counseling and comforting about. This is a normal human reaction. (Even pediatricians, especially when they first start practice, congregate in the corridors of the clinic and hospital, to share confidences and to surreptitiously ask questions without seeming to be too ignorant.)

In our industrial societies there are few extended families and there is very little sense of community, at least in large cities. Parents, especially in the beginning, have a great need just to talk about their babies. But if you require them to make an appointment, pay good money that they need for other purposes, you interfere with this process. We need in our kind of society much more opportunity for counseling without having to go through too many formalities.

I think the 3–4–5 year-old period, in contrast, is one of the most delicious for parents. It's not that there are no problems, but, during this period, children are trying hard to copy their parents all day long, because they admire and love them. If you can't enjoy your children at 3, 4 and 5 years of age, you might as well give them away because it gets progressively harder after the age of 6.

I would underline the need, even in an advanced, rich country like the United States, for day care centers, as more and more mothers go to work. I believe that mothers have as much right as fathers to go to work if they want to, but that the society should be obligated to provide not only adequate day care centers but good ones – especially good ones for families who are otherwise disadvantaged. In the United States we have shamefully few day care centers, and these few are being pinched and squeezed all the time as municipalities get into more and more financial trouble and as President Carter saves more and more money for the Defense Department.

Now at somewhere around 6 years begins a new stage of assertion of independence. The rebellion doesn't go very deep. The child doesn't rebel against the parents' religion or the parents' politics, or the parents' morality. What they rebel against is table manners and cleanliness, and in some ways I think this is more irritating. Instead of wanting to be like their parents, they are watching their peers and trying to be as like them as possible: rough language, dirty old clothes, the hairstyles that are popular in their gang. At meal time the child is kicking the leg of the table all through the meal. But, when the mother says, "Stop it!" the child, in surprise, asks, "What was I doing?" The child's antagonism is veiled from the child. Children argue. They balk every night against going to bed on time. They pit their teachers against their parents. My oldest son, when he was around 8 or 9, asked one day, "Which is bigger, red blood cells or white blood cells?" I fell in to the trap of thinking that he was appealing to my wisdom. I said, "White blood cells, of course," and he said, "Oh, no they aren't. Our science teachers says that red blood cells are bigger." I kept wondering why he was picking fights with me. Later, I realized that the child's need is to get the parent down off a pedestal. The desire is so great that his ears prick up when he hears the teacher talking about *anything* that might be used at home. And he will, without realizing it, turn upside down what the teachers say in order to start an argument at home.

Now I want to talk about the importance of good schools, of which there are too few. There are several serious errors that schools and universities tend to slip into. One is to emphasize memorization: the assumption that if you have memorized something, that means you have some kind of wisdom whether it's drill, definitions, rules, or the teacher's opinions. We have to have some of these preliminaries to education, but it's totally wrong to think of these as being the essence of education. Another bad thing that schools do is to require that each child keep in step with the rest of the class, instead of seeing that the purpose should be to bring each individual to greater maturity. If you are a 7-year old, you have to conform to second grade standards; and the teacher will report you to your parents if you do not.

There are two perspectives I find helpful in trying to keep straight what education should be. One is to think what education is in societies that don't have formal schooling. Girls and boys begin their education by playing at being women and men, with dolls, pots and pans, pretend bows and arrows or fish nets. Then at an appropriate age the boy is allowed to begin to really assist his father; in some societies that's as early as 8 or 9 years of age. Girls are actually taking care of their younger siblings by the age of 5. Young children learn through emotional identification with their parents. They want most of all to grow up and be magnificent people as they imagine their parents are magnificent.

I think that the best education in our formal schools and universities is on the basis of identification, too; and a child can't identify with a teacher unless the teacher is a friendly person. I don't mean *just* friendly, because I've been fascinated with how scornful children are of a teacher who is too easy on them and doesn't challenge them. They say, "She's nice, but she doesn't teach you anything."

John Dewey believed that a child learns not by memorizing, but by doing. This should be the basic principle at all levels of education. In medical education we can see very clearly which approaches are valuable and which ones fail. Since the last part of the nineteenth century we've depended upon the library, the laboratory and text books, and we still have to have these. But it's been known since the beginnings of medicine that basically it must be learned through apprenticeship in practice. Students have to spend months and years seeing patients with an instructor leaning over their shoulder who is pointing out gaps and mis-interpretations in their histories and examinations, discrepancies in their laboratory procedures.

We have also learned, especially around the turn of the century, that medical education must be by feeling, too. When bacteriology, physiology, biochemistry and pathology developed in the last part of the nineteenth century, we had for the first time definite underpinnings for medicine, and specifically for diagnosis. But the result of this emphasis on science was that medicine became ashamed of diagnosing anything that couldn't be demonstrated at the autopsy table or in the laboratory. We lost contact with the vast area of psychosomatic medicine and we lost sensitivity to the doctor-patient relationship. By about 1925 we had forgotten that patients were human beings and had feelings.

Now to turn all this into recommendations: I think that in elementary school, in high school, in the undergraduate years in the university and in graduate studies, students should be learning primarily by doing. Then they should get together with teachers in class rooms to discuss the significance of what they have actually experienced. Too often we fill our students' minds with concepts and then it is hard for them to get around the concepts and discover what life and people are really like. At the elementary level, children can learn arithmetic by running a school store. Instead of studying arithmetic as a separate subject, writing as a separate subject, reading as a separate subject, geography as a separate subject. American third graders can study American Indians, who naturally fascinate 8 years olds. Then they learn to count like the Indians. They read books about the Indians. They paint murals and make models of Indian villages. At the university level, we should have many practicums. Everybody should have to be working with people in some field or another, preferably in the field that they expect to enter. Then they should come back and discuss in the class or the conference room what has been experienced.

All the way through we should put an emphasis on learning by feeling. At the elementary level, when two children get into a fight, the teacher can step in, not to say, "No! No! you naughty children," but to lead a discussion of how the fight got started, and how the feelings got involved. She can get into subjects like religion, prejudices, and racial prejudices.

Sex education should not be taught by the gym department as if it were a muscle, or by the school physician or the school nurse as if it were a disease. Sex is a part of everything. It has to do with poetry, it has to do with history. When high school students are studying the "Idylls of the King", they should be not only allowed but encouraged, to bring the discussion back to their own lives and problems. When children find that their teacher is a wise and understanding person, they will gradually bring into the classroom discussions more and more of their feelings and concerns.

How do you recruit mature teachers who can comfortably discuss these real aspects of life? Part of the answer is to give enough money to the schools so that the schools can have small classes and so that schools can select mature people to be teachers. We have in the United States a recurring battle in education in which the conservatives say, "Let's get back to the basics!" Basics means reading, writing and arithmetic only. These conservatives say, "Let's get rid of the frills!" There are people in all societies, in all nations, who think if we could just get back to the good old days, as they remember them when they were children, everything would be all right.

I believe that there should be discussions of family life, life adjustment, marriage, career choices, driver education. More deaths of adolescents and youths are caused by poor driving habits than by any other cause.

I think that if law schools had more concern for learning by doing and by feeling, it would be easier for me to talk to my lawyer. Theologians should be studying human relations as well as theology. I think that even engineering students should be studying people's feelings, because they'll have to deal with feelings too.

Now I have a more basic complaint about schools and universities. Most of them are teaching compliance with the society as it exists. If you don't believe that, find out what happens to teachers who try to bring up dangerous topics such as socialism. We are teaching students all the way through, in all but the very best schools, to be good, to be quiet, to pay attention to what is being taught so that they will be able to fit into one of the slots that their society has prepared for them. Now this might not be so bad if a society had solved its major problems: but the society I live in is getting into deeper trouble all the time. We have unnecessary poverty. We have no health insurance for all our people. We have racial prejudice still searing the souls of black children and of other minorities, giving them feelings of inadequacy, that will hound them the rest of their lives. We should be encouraging a questioning, skeptical attitude on the part of our students. We should be encouraging initiative. We should be encouraging creativity and new ways of thinking about things. Our children, instead of learning the ridiculous half truths and untruths they are taught in civics classes about how our government is meant to function, should learn how Government really operates. They should go to City Hall to discuss with the Mayor and other officials some of the city's persistent problems and then get back into class to discuss frankly the issues and the competence of the officials.

Good for children in the adolescent years to go and see the horrible handling – or rather mishandling – of delinquents.

We deprive our children at the high school level by giving them no opportunity to do real work or to identify with adults. We keep our children and young people in a separate group, without dignity or acknowledged worth.

The needs of adolescents and youths are increasingly complex, especially in a rapidly changing industrial society; but they are offered, at least in the United States, no framework of spiritual values to guide them.

I believe that human beings are potentially materialistic, but also potentially spiritual. They need to find a meaning in life, and feel stranded without it. Some of our youths are turning to eastern mystical religions, having received no comfort from their parents' churches. At least we could give them a sense of obligation about serving their fellow humans.

One of the things that makes being a parent of adolescents nowadays so particularly difficult is the independent mindedness of young people. This is a remarkable change from that time of my youth. A few years ago at Western Reserve Medical School, I tried to intimidate the first year class because so many of them in the first month of school were coming late to lectures. Then they began bringing coffee in cardboard cups. At first, they took surreptitious sips of coffee and hid the cup; but as time went on, they became bolder and they finally reached a stage where they would keep the cup at their lips all through the lecture, nursing it gently. You got the feeling, as lecturer, that they were looking scornfully at you over the brims of their cups, as if to say, "What crap". I asked them politely to come on time or not come at all. This didn't make the slightest difference. When I myself next had the chance to lecture, I raised my voice and thundered just a little. It was enough to raise goose flesh on my own spine, because it was not usual for a professor to shout at students. I thought that this would surely intimidate them. Not at all. Just as many came late. Then in January they sent an official delegation to my office to complain that the course had no content – the course that I was so proud of, that previous classes loved, and subsequent classes loved – the most insulting thing that you can say to an instructor. I had tried to intimidate them and I had failed utterly, but they intimidated me. I was afraid the dean would hear that they were complaining. I was even more afraid that the rest of the faculty would hear that they were complaining.

This was so different from when I was in medical school. If a lowly instructor scowled with one eyebrow, little waves of anxiety went through the class. They would huddle in the hall and wonder what the instructor was angry about. I think that the difference in young people today is not that they are rude, it's that they don't have antennae out to sense the attitude of the adults that they deal with. I was acutely conscious of my parents' attitude about everything I did. I was scared of every teacher, and of the policeman on the block. I think the basic reason why today's youths can't be intimidated is because they weren't intimidated when they were small children. And that, I think, is because parents now have more trust in their children. They believe Freud, they believe John Dewey, they believe Spock, that children have strong motivation within themselves to mature, to become more grown up and responsible.

I was angry that I couldn't intimidate the medical students. Then I had to retire for reasons of age in 1967 and, because of circumstances, I became a full-time opponent of the war in Vietnam. This time I was delighted by the fact that youths couldn't be intimidated by the federal government, by the universities, by their parents. Since we have so many problems, it's good that young people feel free to make up their own minds and refuse to be intimidated. I only wish there were more activists. The activism that was such a dramatic part of youthful behavior back in the late '60s and early '70s has largely disappeared.

I feel that students at the high school and college years are assailed with many doubts, that they have too many choices to make and too few influences to guide them. I think that parents should be encouraged to express their views on life, even their views on morality (which is not usual today). It's not that youths will obey their parents; we all remember from our own adolescence that we disobeyed when we thought we could get away with it, or thought we were justified. But I think that young people still want to hear what older people believe about life, even if they want to reject these views, then they will at least know what they are rejecting. I believe that they want to hear about spiritual values and moral positions, not only from their parents but from their instructors in the university. This is why, I think, so many students in recent years complain that the university is too impersonal. Universities are still scared of the olden days, when they were dominated by the churches. Teachers feel they mustn't bring their personal views into the class room, that this would be slightly indecent as well as unacademic. But I think students *should* hear the opinions of their instructors. There used to be no fear that they are going to take them lying down. I will end up by saying that in the United States, at least, we are not doing right by children and youths. In fact, we are not doing right by people generally. Government is primarily responsive to industry because of industry's financial contributions to election campaigns. People's needs come second. Another sorry aspect of political life in America is that less than half the people bother to vote and this is very alarming to me. This invites special interest groups to take over the government more and more.

Our government is spending now a hundred and thirty billion dollars a year on more arms when we've got enough now to destroy everybody in the world many times over. We go through a charade like the Salt II talks, as if that was going to bring about a reduction. It has nothing to do with reduction. It's simply an agreement between the defense departments of the United States and the USSR to put a mild limit on further expansion of arms. Meanwhile, cities like New York, Cleveland, and Detroit have gone bankrupt. The governments of those cities can't decide what they should do. They have to ask the bankers for permission. The federal budget, the provisions for health, education, housing and welfare are being progressively squeezed. This is outrageous. It's indecent. Citizens should rouse themselves from their apathy. We have enough resources, enough education in the developed countries to provide a good life for everybody in the world, and we ought to be working for that. There might be some point in piling up arms if they gave security. They don't give any security. Gradually the nuclear arms are spreading to more and more nations and this increases the likelihood of some nuclear disaster, either through brinkmanship, insanity or accident. It's time for professional people to take public stands – as groups and as individuals – since they will be listened to more seriously than some other groups in the community. They should be crying from the house tops: "Let us use our resources for the benefit of people, starting with our children."

Former Professor of Child Development,
Western Reserve University,
Cleveland, Ohio.

Mrs. EDDAH GACHUKIA, M.P. (Kenya)

ATTAINING THE FULL POTENTIAL OF HUMAN ACHIEVEMENT – PHYSICAL, SOCIAL AND PSYCHOLOGICAL

INTRODUCTION

Kenya today is internationally recognized as a rapidly developing country. This new status which our country has been accorded is no doubt due to the Kenya Government's commitment towards the provision of basic services for its population thereby contributing in a significant way to the improvement of the quality of life in the country. It is also due to the peace and stability that has prevailed in Kenya over the last fifteen years. The effort of government, the spirit and practice of Harambee*, that became the development motto of Kenya since independence and the support of friendly countries everywhere account in large measure for the success that Kenya can claim today. And while we in Kenya are flattered that the world has removed us from the list of the least developed countries, we are only too well aware of the long way we still have to go before we can even begin to claim developed status in terms of wide coverage and especially of equitable distribution of basic services. For this surely must be the yardstick by which we can measure our success and our development today.

We know that it is easy for the government and organizations to establish institutions such as schools and training centres, hospitals and health centres, maternal child-health and family planning clinics, adult education classes and even recreation facilities. It is, however, one thing to provide these facilities and another to get the population to identify with them and to utilize them. It is one thing to establish an ideal and even to plan for its achievement. The plan, no matter how elaborate must, however, never be used as the measure of the achievement of that ideal. Rather we must clearly establish how we wish to evaluate our success. For the developing countries to be able to evaluate their achievements meaningfully, it is the contention of this paper that *effective and quality services* have to be provided.

So, to take one aspect of children's development, it is not how many nursery schools and day centres we have established in Kenya that will count. Rather it is the number of Kenyan children who need the services of a nursery school or day care center – the number that are in fact catered to, and the quality control that can be exercised in the establishment and maintenance of these institutions. These are the issues that count. It is our contention that development should not

* Harambee is a collective, cooperative effort by the people to help themselves "putting or pooling (resources) together – supplementing government effort in an effort to hasten development".

S. H. Fine, R. Krell, and Tsung-yi Lin (Eds.), 'Today's Priority in Mental Health' 15–24.

be measured in terms of how many child-health centres we have constructed in the last fifteen years, but rather the number of children provided for, other medical services available from these clinics, the personnel we employ, and the quality of services rendered that must determine the pace of upward mobility in Kenya's ability to adequately meet the development needs of her children.

Observed from this angle of qualitative evaluation, "developmental needs" of Kenyan children become typical of any developing country – sharing with other African countries the problems of under-development due to lack of resources, inadequacy of qualified personnel and lack of awareness – all factors that are crucial hindrances to development. The rapid socio-economic changes that have taken place in our societies, up-rooting and undermining traditional practices, cause many African nations to find themselves overtaken by events and unable to cope with the new situation that has arisen. Such fundamental issues of socio-economic nature like the rural/urban migration, land consolidation and the introduction of the institution of formal education as the gauge for individual personal development, have their varied effects on the living patterns of the people and especially on the established patterns of traditional family life, child rearing and the division of labour. Besides these factors, developing countries share, in varied degrees the inability to provide a minimum and equitable level of development because we in Kenya inherited a system that was organized on racial lines and geographical uneveness, and this has been difficult to overcome despite our commitment to African socialism. Even the gauges that we have for evaluating development in any given area have been found inadequate at the national level. In considering 'developmental needs' of children in a country like Kenya, therefore, one needs to go beneath the surface of structure, institutions and ideals, to discover the true situation of specific groups and individuals and their peculiar needs. Only then can one identify those who form the target groups and who urgently need help.

Although our frame of reference is that of the Kenyan experience, we feel that some of the issues we intend to pursue in our discussion are also relevant to other developing countries even if there may exist some degree of variation in their quality and coverage.

We shall now look at a number of areas related to the developmental needs of children and families based on the Kenyan experience. Numerous factors contributing to mental, physical and emotional development of children are inter-related and we propose to discuss them as follows:

1. PRE-NATAL NEEDS

Many of our children are underprivileged during pre-natal life because of the general nutritional status of the mother. This situation will persist for as long as our social welfare system makes no provision for basic requirements for mothers-to-be. When we consider that with the gradual breakdown of traditional

African extended family systems, mothers-to-be and new mothers have become increasingly deprived, lacking as they do the supportive services of their own mothers, grandmothers, sisters, aunts and age-groups, mothers-to-be continue to labour and carry the heavy burdens of African rural life so much so that a great number of children are born prematurely without the necessary precautions for their survival (Kenyatta 1961, Fox 1967). Because of their pre-occupation with and involvement in the hazards of everyday life in providing for the basic needs of their families, expectant mothers neglect their own nutritional needs even where food is plentiful. The pre-natal development of the baby thus directly suffers. Many young mothers, even those who have attained formal education are unable to relate their feeding habits to the growth of their unborn child. Few are aware of the requirements for special organs, such as for brain growth. Most traditional systems emphasized quality food after childbirth but not during pregnancy.

2. POST-NATAL NEEDS

(a) *Modern Maternity Expertise*

The fact that a good number of our babies continue to be born outside areas where there is *modern maternity expertise* means that complications resulting from prolonged labour, lack of oxygen, infections and other problems related to childbirth continue to add to the numbers of children born with varying disabilities. The lack of maternal and baby clinics within the reach of most mothers results in diseases and infections remaining undetected and thereby unattended. It is depressing to learn that the majority of cases that account for the rising number of disabled children in many developing countries could have been prevented or successfully treated in their early stages. We need to give local traditional midwives hygienic tools and basic knowledge.

(b) *High Infant Mortality*

The high rate of infant mortality is another common disaster that affects family life in a fundamental way. Brought up within a culture where the primary purpose of marriage is procreation, and where the perpetuation of the family line is still greatly valued, the young mother resists family planning that advocates no child-bearing. Social customs and taboos that facilitated the spacing of children are no longer operative and so, her resistance to family planning results in frequent pregnancies – the consequences are harmful to both herself and her children.

(c) *Education*

It is becoming increasingly unrealistic for African nations to hedge around the problems affecting the care of the pre-school child by insisting that the African extended family system takes care of that. Indeed it was rural mothers themselves who in Kenya recognized that because of land consolidation (which separated families), constant family and individual migration and the growth of primary education, they needed a place they could leave their children in safety while they went about their many and varied tasks.

The pattern of development in most countries is going to rely more on new relationships and forms of societal organizations in supporting the mother in child care, and not on the cherished system of the extended family. The idea of day-care centre or nursery school is attractive to many parents and especially mothers because it carries with it the magic of education – laying the foundation for formal schooling. Unfortunately, few of the so-called day-care centres or nursery schools are as yet organized in a way that they provide the care and security that could substitute for mother or other members of the family. Nor do they provide an environment that would motivate the young child, stimulating him in personality development and creativity. Experience of some of these institutions leads one to believe that these children would be better off running after goats and cows or skidding in the mud after the rains.

A recent study carried out in nursery schools in Nairobi revealed extreme situations where in some privately owned expensive nursery schools, the children had an ideal atmosphere with pleasant stimulating surroundings, lots of challenging equipment, adequate expert teachers and nurses to care for the children – about 12–15 children per teacher – even meals thrown into the bargain. These children have regular medical checks. Nursery schools in this category were found to be more responsive to the creative and aesthetic needs of the child. The other extreme belongs to Harambee nursery schools built by parents who cannot afford to send their children to even the Local Authority nursery schools, but who nevertheless find the idea of 'school' an attractive alternative to leaving children roaming the streets while they are at work. One such school in Mathare, the slum area of Nairobi, had over 75 children in one class manned by an untrained teacher. The building was poorly constructed and had inadequate ventilation. The grounds reflected the general standard of the slum village – pools of stagnant water and garbage. One wondered how such an environment of squalor could be converted into an area for human productivity. No meals are served here and the children undergo no medical attention as their school is outside the control of the City health authorities. This category of nursery school comprised 70 schools out of a total of 215 (about 35%). Of the 14 791 children attending nursery schools in Nairobi, over 5000 attended one such school (Gakuru, In Press). There was a great emphasis on numeracy and literacy – work that the children were clearly not ready for. All they could do was to 'parrot' what their 'teacher' said.

The majority of nursery schools in the rural areas lack stimulation. The "teachers" in such schools are barely trained and so have no means of detecting emotional and physical needs of the children under their care. If a child has difficulties performing tasks assigned to him, he is punished rather than helped to overcome them. Even when reading and writing difficulties are identified, the teachers do not have adequate knowledge of or facilities for corrective measures. A national health service for all children attending all nursery and primary schools regardless of status, is recommended. Currently, even in the most advanced sectors like the Nairobi City Council, such services cover only children in public schools and are non-existent for children in primvate Harambee schools where the majority of the needy children are.

Recently, the Kenya Government introduced a national milk program to all primary schools – a most commendable effort even though still in its infancy. National programs do, however, tend to overlook the real target – in this case, the hungry and malnourished. This is because such programs cover both the needy and those who do not need essential supplements like milk. Indications from this particular program are that those schools within the regions with better communication get easily covered while remote areas with bad roads cannot be reached. As it happens, it is the children in remote areas who need milk more.

Research in education has established that the social background and especially home environment of a child eventually makes a remarkable impact on his education. Nevertheless, a tug-of-war exists between parents and teachers as to who is responsible for what. Who exactly is to blame for any visible shortcomings in the child's performance? For a long time, however, the school has deliberately presented the child with a novel environment and experience that was totally different from the home environment. It was commonly believed by colonialist educators that the African home had nothing to offer to the child's school learning. Even the medium of instruction had to be English which made the child's experiences prior to coming to school irrelevant. Experiencing this discrepancy between the school and the home, parents feel inadequate to help their children and are excited to hear their children speak a language they themselves do not know, little realizing the crucial relationship that exists between language and concept-development. At Independence, it was the parents who insisted that English continue to be the medium of instruction right from Primary One. Fluency in and knowledge of English continues to account, in large measure, for the Kenyan student's academic achievement. Because of this feeling of inadequacy by parents in matters concerning the children's academic work, the overall developmental needs of the child have tended to be left increasingly in the hands of the teacher. Parents are only too happy to surrender their responsibilities submitting to the 'mysteries' of a new world that the teacher is able to unfold for their children.

Unfortunately for the primary school child, this uncertainty as to who is responsible, especially for the personal development of the child, leaves a vacuum in matters of personal relationships and especially in the area of sex education, which in the traditional set-up was thoroughly taught during the initiation period

(Kenyatta 1961, Mbiti 1969). Gaps left by the school are only identified long after the problem has gotten out of hand.

In the primary school, the teachers, despite their training, are unable to recognize children's developmental needs. A child who has problems is easily dubbed backward and condemned to the 'slow' learner's group for all time. Some classes are so large (45–60 children) that no individual attention to the child's needs can be expected. Difficulties in reading and writing, especially in the foreign language are common and they are transferred to other areas of learning that require these skills. Such difficulties are reflected in the child's performance at public examinations which are the crucial determinants of the child's whole future. The high rate of drop-out for girls in upper primary and secondary schools due to teenage pregnancies is one clear case of neglect by both home and school, each one failing to recognize its role in the dual responsibility for the development of the child. It is also due to the cultural conflict that has arisen in our society. Traditional values clash with modern values while the society has not yet evolved workable and acceptable ethical standards for all its members. In this situation, the children suffer most as they get confused by the double standards displayed by the adults.

The urban environment has opened up a whole new world for children in the way of films, literature and other media. Children are on one hand exposed to a wide field of experience while, at the same time, the adult world frustrates them by wishing to dictate what they should or should not know. This state of affairs results in serious conflicts and problems for the adolescents and teenagers. This is the so-called generation gap.

3. PARENT-CHILD RELATIONSHIP

(a) *The mother*

The full awareness of the mother of the needs of the child is fundamental. It is an issue to which developing nations must give priority. The socio-economic conditions of individual families may not allow for the proper feeding of young children, even where food is available. It is also not certain that mothers are consciously aware of the minimum nutritional needs of the child. Since the majority of mothers continue to breast-feed their babies, more so in the rural areas, the weaning period becomes the crucial issue when considering problems of undernourishment and malnutrition. In quite a few societies, children were weaned almost overnight on 'soft' food that is not the best for growing children, e.g. bananas, potatoes and maize porridge. The shift from traditional to modern farming has also affected the food situation in a negative manner. Sorghum, millet, *Wimbi* and other grains that formed the staple diet for porridge and *Ugali* and which were more nutritious than the popular maize meal, have almost disappeared. The introduction of cash-crops such as coffee, tea and pyrethrum has caused the reduction of growing legumes and grains which are the commonest sources of proteins and vitamins. Although it could be argued that the cash obtained from cash crops is used to buy items that supplement the family diet, it has been found that the family fails to purchase the vital foodstuffs such as eggs, milk, beans and vegetables.

The awareness of the mother must, however, go beyond the domain of nutrition. The immunization of young babies is one phenomenon the mother must be taught to understand and adhere to. A number of illnesses, particularly those related to diarrhoea continue to take their toll on the health of the young child. The mother needs to be brought closer to the world of simple medicine to recognize that all diarrhoea is not related to "teething" and that given proper hygienic conditions, she can eliminate such common illnesses. Again we emphasize, it is not enough to build health centres and to stock them and staff them. It is more important that parents and particularly mothers be made to realize the usefulness of such facilities. The authorities should see health centres not merely as places of curing but more as centres for disseminating information on preventive measures. Because of the general state of poor health existing in some places, parents are slow in identifying the degree of children's illnesses. There are far too many cases of mothers going out to work only to come back home to find seriously ill children when they thought all the child was suffering from was a simple cold. Where baby and maternal clinics exist and the population does not make full use of them, it could be due to attitudes, distance and the time-tables. The timing is especially important considering that mothers have to fit in visits to such clinics within their heavy daily schedules.

The role of women within the family has tended to become more onerous as developing countries continue to develop. The awareness of the mother concerning good hygiene in the home for instance leads the mother to need more water for cleaning and other domestic use. This means she has to travel more times to and from the river to fetch water. Her awareness leads her to new ventures and new responsibilities (e.g. growing more crops, keeping poultry or cows). Her workload continues to increase and she has less time to spend with her child. The older children that used to assist her in looking after the baby and in other simple tasks around the home are all in school. Mother and baby are, therefore, deprived of the traditional help. For the sake of the development of the child in the early stages, therefore, developing nations need to constantly evaluate the role of the mother and to take measures that will ensure that she is not so much over-burdened with work that she has no time to attend to the needs of her child. Such measures as the provision of clean water in or near the home go a long way towards alleviating the heavy work women have to do and thus allow more time for them to attend to the needs of their families.

The situation of the mother in paid employment is critical in the sense that she cannot regulate her work-load in order to suit even the barest needs of her child. Unlike the conditions prevailing in developed countries, the working mother in Kenya often has no alternative but to go out to work. The child is frequently left in hands of inexperienced girls (*Ayas*) who cannot maintain the standard of baby care that the mother would like her child to have. Kenya grants only two months paid maternity leave to nursing mothers. The mother can of course take unpaid leave to breast-feed her baby but this she would do at the risk of losing her job which many cannot afford to do because of their economic status and the needs of the nation. The establishment of good day-care centres is relevant here as is the proper training of *mature* women who can then be employed to assist working mothers.

(b) *The Father*

The absence of the father is one factor many families have to contend with. It is also no longer practical to assume that in the absence of the father, an uncle or some other male member in the immediate family circle will fulfill the role of the father. Traditionally, although the father played a rather peripheral role during early childhood, he did take over the education and upbringing of his sons soon after the age of five or six. The clear division of labour between men and women made this delineation of responsibilities between fathers and mothers in the task of child-rearing straightforward (Kenyatta 1961). With the emergence of the nuclear family, however, and the constant absence of the father, usually working away from home, the role of the father within the family has diminished. The role of the father within the family in the new changing environment needs to be urgently reviewed and evaluated to enable him to contribute more positively to his children's development. In many instances, the father acquired more in the way of formal education than the mother. The knowledge thus gained can be used to the benefit of the whole family. Many girls and especially boys identify increasingly more with the career world of their fathers. Due to lack of higher education, the mother's world of work even if she is a professional, is not as varied or attractive to youngsters as that of the father. This calls for greater participation of the father in the upbringing of the child.

African literature depicting life in the traditional African homestead portrays the father as the pillar of stability and peace in the home (Ngugi, 1961). The social change that has taken place in our society caused by external factors and intervention by foreign cultures has affected the family significantly. The father who is faced with unemployment and has no land, yet has a large family, cannot possibly be the pillar of strength around which the family thrives.

4. ASSESSMENT

How shall we assess the development of our children and society? Education in developing countries is highly prized as an opening to economic security and social success. It is important, therefore, to urgently develop assessment tools in this area so as to ensure that we measure the full potential of our children and not only their success in academic achievement. The current measures of assessment, be they in the way of IQ Tests or national examinations, are influenced by the culture of the child. Such testing systems favor the urban child and disregard the early experiences of the rural child. This obviously puts the rural child at a disadvantage from the very beginning. The tremendously varied background and experience of the Kenyan child demands that valid tests for various groups and geographical environments be devised. It is crucial that we devise tests that depict the African child's own background.

Developing countries lack qualified manpower in this crucial area and urgently need the assistance of educators, psychologists and social scientists to fill this vacuum. Countries that suffer from shortages of basic essentials like food, drugs and water cannot be expected to place the development of psychometric tools as a priority.

5. THE PLACE OF THE HANDICAPPED

The handicapped children in our societies are products of the socio-economic conditions we have tried to describe above. Some of their disabilities result from problems of under-development, pre-natal and post-natal negligence, natural disasters, lack of awareness, disease or absolute deprivation. They are, nevertheless, rightful members of our societies deserving similar, if not greater, attention to that given to other children. Yet it has been argued that since developing countries cannot even meet the basic needs of 'normal' children, why bother about the handicapped? This attitude accounts for the common negligence by developing countries in establishing facilities for the handicapped. The whole social system needs orientation towards sympathetic consideration for the plight of the handicapped and mentally ill. Sympathy for the handicapped has to be learned, as traditionally, such children were treated as cursed and were made to suffer contempt and ridicule. Parents with disabled children should be identified and helped to better understand their children so that they can present them for any available services.

Previously, the care and education of the disabled were left almost entirely in the hands of NGO's (National Government Officers). It is gratifying to note that from 1979, the Kenya Government intends to take over the financial burden of running schools and training institutions for the disabled and to assist the NGO's with the training of personnel for this area. It is crucial that the handicapped take their place within their society, learning skills that will ensure their survival.

We have endeavoured to demonstrate that the developmental needs of children in developing countries remain largely unfulfilled. A lot of human potential that is crucial for development remains, therefore, untapped and underdeveloped. We would like to make the following recommendations:

1. National development plans and welfare systems need to be oriented towards the real areas of need.
2. The meagre resources of developing countries should be utilized in a manner that ensures a more equitable distribution which is a prerequisite for true and meaningful development.

3. Parents and especially mothers should be educated and their roles evaluated in the light of the rapid social change.

4. The quality of day-care centres and nursery school education needs urgent improvement.

5. More and deliberate measures should be taken at the national and individual level to ensure care of the disabled.

6. School curriculum and assessment tools need to reflect the child's environment rather than uproot him entirely from his socio-cultural experience.

7. A national health service covering all pre-school and primary school children is necessary.

8. Research should be undertaken to discover what percentage of the child population is not covered by government programs and why.

Member of Parliament,
President of National Council of Women,
Nairobi,
Kenya

REFERENCES

Fox, L. (ed.)
1967 East African Childhood: Three Versions. Nairobi: Oxford University Press.

Gakuru, O. N.
Pre-School Education and Access to Educational Opportunities, (In Press).

Kenyatta, J.
1961 Facing Mount Kenya. London: Secker & Warburg.

Mbiti, J.
1969 African Religions and Philosophy. Heinemann.

Ngugi, J.
1962 Weep Not, Child. Heinemann (African Writers' Series).

1979–1983 Development Plan
1979 Nairobi: Government Printer.

Dr. SERGE LEBOVICI (France)

THE NEEDS OF THE CHILD AND HIS DEVELOPMENT

When we examine the development of the child, we generally assume that it depends on biological, social and psychological factors which we readily represent in the form of a pyramid with the psychological factors occurring at the top. It seems to me that this metaphor does not reflect reality, which is infinitely more complex, and that the interweaving of biological, social and psychological factors must be emphasized at the outset. To demonstrate this, I will mention just one example: it has to do with the birth of a smile.

We are well aware that mothers, when they obseve the faces made by their babies, imagine that the child is smiling at them, whereas this is not the case at all and that the grimaces formed by his mouth are only the expression of an archaic reflex which will later disappear, the bucco-lingual orientation reflex. It is, however, on the basis of this reflex that, at a fairly imprecise date – let us say around the sixth week – a smile occurs specifically in response to the approach of a human face, which is producing sounds and is seen head-on by the child. The child's smile when he sees his mother's face presupposes the existence of this archaic reflex, and the meaning given it by the mother. This example is entirely typical of the interweaving of biological, psychological and social factors, and is typical of the type of thing implied by the environment's intervention into the genetic program for the child's development.

It is appropriate to study the development of the child in relation to the mother's reactions, and I shall do so by examining how the satisfaction or lack of satisfaction of the child's needs, have a bearing on the mental functions of the mother. As regards the child, we can assume two fundamental principles in order to understand his development. One is the state of absolute dependence in which he finds himself; the other is his ability to master exteroceptive or interoceptive stimulation by various discharges. In other words, as daily experience shows us, the newborn infant is protected against stimulation. But at the same time, and this is what ensures him of this protection, he forms almost a single unit with his mother. It is within the framework of this unit formed by the newborn infant and his mother's care that his needs are satisfied, essentially those which bring him peace, which concern food, cleanliness and comfort. All of the experiences thus stored will be of use to the child increasingly as mother's care diminishes. By learning, at first by chance, to stimulate the erogenous zones, the child will thus be able to recreate for himself and by himself the pleasure attached to memory traces. When the baby happens by chance to put his finger in his mouth, he sucks on it as if nursing. Thus he stimulates the oral area which extends far beyond the mucous membranes of the lips, mouth and pharynx to

S. H. Fine, R. Krell, and Tsung-yi Lin (Eds.), 'Today's Priorities in Mental Health' 25–29.

include that part of the body which involves the muscular activity from the head to the tips of his fingers, as when he holds his mother's fingers while being fed his meal. By sucking his finger, which he put into his mouth by chance, or by nursing without sucking his finger, the child thereby rediscovers all the pleasurable experiences which he acquired.

In times of mother's absence, when his needs are not being satisfied, the child learns to hallucinate satisfaction and to recreate in a very rudimentary form the agent of sedation, his mother. To use Freudian terminology, we can return to a metaphor of his, in *Three Essays on the Theory of Sexuality*, that the breast is born of the absence of the breast. In other words, the sequence is one of desire being supported by need; and of the satisfaction of desire depending first upon the hallucination of pleasure, then upon hallucination of the object.

In turn, the mother can be recreated only because she has existed. The existing mother is one who not only institutes herself as the mother of a child who is real, but also the child which she makes up out of her fantasies and imagination. When she was pregnant the mother began to build up a symbiotic system with this child whose life and whose movements she could feel. The desire for a child is obviously extremely complex, and along with other factors is complicated by the mother's own conflicts with her personal environment, including the child's father and her own parents. The extent to which she identifies with her own mother and to which oedipal desires are rekindled in the course of her relationship with her husband and in the course of her pregnancy, intervene to give the imaginary child some of his traits.

For an example we need only to remember the ways in which children's names are chosen. Naturally, in many civilizations cultural or religious traditions intervene to determine the child's name, but in many western countries the choice of name is often a response to this imaginary child. Sometimes it is the name of a dead relative who is missed and whose memory the name is meant to rekindle. In other instances it is the name of some hero who played an important role in the childhood of the father or the mother. In the same way, the sex first chosen often indicates the mother's preferences and those of her husband.

After the delivery, the narcissistic fulfillment which was one of the motivations for pregnancy is called into question by the reality of a child which the mother often doesn't know how to handle. Her inability to give the child basic care is often striking and it makes her feel helpless at a time when, for all sorts of reasons, she may be experiencing a period of depression. The usefulness of this depression has been convincingly demonstrated by Winnicott, in his description of the primary maternal concern which causes the mother to be entirely at the disposal of the child, after which she separates herself from him little by little. There are conflicts which the mother endures between her period of narcissistic expansiveness during pregnancy and her depressed feeling of emptiness after the birth.

Given these conditions, the mother's ability to fulfill her task, to respond to the child's needs, and to separate herself from him gradually in order to return to her normal family life imply a whole series of vicissitudes which are resolved by the child's progress and his ability to hallucinate pleasure and, consequently, to function mentally. These are the contradictory bases upon which the modes of interaction between mother and child are founded.

One such interaction relates to the eye contact which is so fundamentally important and which involves a considerable reciprocity of which most people are unaware. To use Winnicott's vivid description, the child looking at his mother must see her, but must also see her looking at him. What the mother expects of her child is more than he is capable of accomplishing and this expectation provides an anticipatory role to his development. In France, this is generally called the mother's creative anticipation which play a fundamental structuring role. In this context the example of the infant's crying out has often been given to emphasize the fact that this manifestation, at first simply a means of expression, becomes a summons because the mother gives it this meaning.

The theory of the child's needs just presented is based essentially on his initial total dependence on his mother's care. The interest in the study of animal behavior by ethologists has led scientists to elaborate the concept of attachment, as John Bowlby has done. The applicability of this concept of attachment to the human child will not be discussed now but ethological experiments are particularly eloquent in this context – not only Harlow's experiments on chimpanzees, but also more recent experiments which demonstrate the constraint imposed by one's first experience of the environment. I will cite only one. In certain black seagulls of Greenland, food is taken by the offspring when he taps on the underside of the beaks of his parents who deposit in his pharynx the food which they were keeping in their mouths. The experimental triggering of behavior in newborn offspring of this species by means of a decoy is very interesting. Two types of decoy can in fact be created, the first consisting of a red strip in the shape of the beak and the second in the form of the black head and red beak. It has been observed that at birth the young are responsive to the red decoy resembling the beak, and that this decoy triggers the movements which normally culminate in the tapping on the underside of the parent's beaks. Beginning with the eighth day the second decoy – the head which was of no interest at birth – achieves its full value, whereas the first decoy – the red beak – loses value. This implies, therefore, that the genetic constraint is strongly reduced and that the complex form eventually intervenes. The initial genetic constraint could be likened to that of a color, red, contrasting with all the black beaks of the parent gulls.

The polarity between dependence and attachment is of specific interest insofar as it concerns the study of the social needs of children. Psychoanalysts have attached particular importance to the role of the mother in their study of the needs of the child. The importance of the mother implies that personal contacts between the baby and his mother should be encouraged, and that social measures should be taken to this end.

If, on the other hand, we incline more to the attachment theory, we will aim at creating a situation in which the child can find satisfaction of his attachment needs, even if these are not directly represented by the mother. It is self-evident that in certain particular social or cultural situations, the attachment theory permits the creation of the most favorable institutional situations. But in any case, when these institutions are created, they must fulfill the requirements implied by the needs which were pointed out earlier, namely that they create multiple and authentic bonds between the child and his environment, which is represented essentially by human beings, especially women, who must be well prepared to play a positive role in relation to young developing babies.

The interactions which have been emphasized lead to the development of the concept of communication, subverbal communication, which is achieved not only by words, even meaningless ones, but also by the body, by rhythms and smells, which then must be followed by verbal communication. The latter is being called into question in urbanized, technological western society where the family has been reduced to the nuclear unit. When we study, for example, the role of the father in the family in industrial society, we find ourselves in a specific situation quite different from the societies of transmission described by Eric Erikson. In these, the little boy is initiated by the adults and the old people. He goes hunting, having made his own bow like his father and using it as he does. How different from the families we know in which children have only a vague notion of the work done by their father, whom they reduce to an anonymous cog in a meaningless technological society.

It is this earlier communication which makes language learning possible, and hence schooling. It would be an illusion, as many of my colleagues have pointed out, to believe that possession of the written language is nothing more than the fruit of school learning. The mother's language, its use and the power that its use confers – this is what can give the child a real taste for learning to read and write.

Consequently progress in education and learning depends on knowledge of the needs of the child. I would like to emphasize the importance of the latency period described by Freud, not in the naive meaning which it is normally given as that of the disappearance of sexual needs, but as the expression of a tremendous effort of repression, an act of making latent, which then permits the child to devote his attention to learning, to acquiring knowledge, and to taking advantage of all these sublimitations. Here again, this individual development must be accompanied by the satisfaction of social needs. Cultural injustices concern the excessively large family in certain underdeveloped nations just as much as they do the reduced family in which the leisure civilization plays a dominant role. Children need stimulating educational institutions at a sufficiently early age. The system of kindergartens and preschools therefore constitutes an absolutely essential requirement in our culture in its present state.

Later comes adolescence, and we could not describe in a few words the needs of this period. I mention it just for the purpose of pointing out that in industrial civilization in its current state, the dependent period of childhood is prolonged by an adolescence during which the learning of a trade or profession has become a lengthy business and in which, at the same time, needs are exacerbated by the requirements of the consumer society. Faced with this conflict, parents have gotten into the habit of hiding by 'counter-identifying with adolescents', or of pretending to be adolescents themselves and thus appearing ridiculous. Parents need to understand and accept their situation. They are aging individuals, losing strength in the eyes of their children, who are indeed capable of taking their place, in their own way. With inherited values they will rebuild their own house stone by stone.

This description of the needs of the child and the developing adolescent is obviously too brief, but it shows the extent of the risks which become evident during the course of his development. Here it is necessary to bring together two concepts: that of vulnerability and that of risk.

In a rather schematic way we can say that vulnerability is the heritage with which the child develops, not only at birth but during his growth. Vulnerability is biological risk. But this biological risk cannot be isolated. For example, there is biologic risk in being the child of psychotic parents, but that also presupposes another type of vulnerability. It has been noted that a very frequent syndrome in children of psychotic parents is to have a difficult birth and to be submitted to inconsistent placements in institutions at an early age. Thus biologic vulnerability cannot be separated from the psychological and social risks which the child faces.

Vulnerability also often exists in places where we do not expect it. Contrary to what is often said, the strong sex is not in fact the male sex, and we know that little boys are much more threatened than little girls on the level of their emotional development as well as on that of their physical growth.

Bearing in mind biological determinants, their risks must be considered in order to apply a specific preventive policy. We know that these risks are particularly important in developing nations, in western nations among immigrant families, and countries where the technological advances are combined with massive unemployment. Can development be ensured simply by the satisfaction of social needs? This is really the question we must ask of ourselves. Is it our role to encourage the creation of special institutions for vulnerable children exposed to multiple risks? Since such institutions are certainly necessary, we should help to define their role and make them as good as possible for the child, and his or her family. But the satisfaction of the elementary needs of the child remains uppermost and we must assist him so that he is capable of facing the difficulties of the environment in which he lives. From this perspective, the notion of competence as it has been popularized in the United States, as meaning not only knowledge, constitutes an absolutely essential goal with regard to the needs of the child. We have shown how these needs depend on the interconnection of biological, social and psychological factors.

Professeur de Psychiatrie de l'Enfant,
L'Université de Paris XIII,
UER Expérimentale de Médecine
et de Biologie Humaine de Bobigny,
Paris, France

SECTION TWO

SOCIETAL CONTEXT

INTRODUCTION

The first section of this book addressed the developmental needs of the child. Such needs intersect at every conceivable phase with the child's environment, familial and societal. The inextricability of mind and body extends as well to individual and society. The interplay between society and person is a theme in Eisenberg's elegant discussion of how culture determines views of who is well and who is sick. Social and societal life influences mankind's biology and psychology and persons decide whether they will be patients or 'ill' according to their expectations of life. The physician's view of illness is not necessarily that which is experienced by patients.

Since the nature of human society influences human biology and human psychology, Eisenberg emphasizes that in preventive approaches, one must come to grips with social determinants. Pertinent to preventive mental health are issues pertaining to early puberty, unwanted pregnancies, abortions, increase in longevity, retirement ages, birth rates, women in the labour force, social mobility and its stresses, the need for people and a social network, and education and its relevance to vocation. Within this social fabric are the various factors which may determine a person's wellness.

Hasan adds a further dimension to the concern we share for the improved and proper application of mental health service to the children of our world. He emphasizes the particular problems of developing countries caught between poverty and deprivation and advanced and advancing technology. For developing nations it is a time of profound and rapid change with the expected consequences of instability. The latter can produce great psychosocial conflict and upheaval, or perhaps provide opportunities for new systems of health care based on an awareness of the process of change.

Hasan discusses some of the effects of major social forces on the development of developing nations: the high proportion of children under age 15 (40% of total population in developing nations), infant mortality (six times that of industrial countries), urbanization as a result of and a factor in poverty, the changing status of women and child rearing, and most importantly, the absence of a social infrastructure necessary to evolve a society with progressive and planned modernization. The author offers suggestions which deserve serious consideration by social planners, politicians, and others empowered to provide services to children and families.

Eisenberg and Hasan both have emphasized the rapidity with which our world is changing. But not withstanding poverty or riches, urban or rural life, technology or primitiveness, it is the cumulative pressure on the family as a unit which has caused the greatest concern.

S. H. Fine, R. Krell, and Tsung-yi Lin (Eds.), 'Today's Priorities in Mental Health' 33–34.

Miller takes the reader back to fundamentals. Given that mankind is better able to provide food, protection and shelter, what will sustain men and women spiritually? The fundamental beliefs in a faith, in the worth of work, in love, are interwoven with civilization, tradition, religion, personal and family values. The rapid erosion of fundamentals, the brittleness of commitments, particularly to family; these are the structural weaknesses upon which societal forces exert relentless pressures. Television educates, not parents alone; young people predominate in families, not the elders; and parents no longer consider their children the only priority. The changes are profound and Miller is appropriately mystified to find that people still feel life is best when with people you love, at a time when, mostly, allegiances to one another, are brief.

Watanabe too finds the world a little mystifying, or at best, imbalanced. He describes the world as 'schizophrenic' since a recent major international congress was devoted to extricating women from their families while the focus in this, the International Year of the Child, is concerned with re-integrating the family as the root of a child's happiness. Watanabe views these trends as incompatible, and that happiness for women cannot be found in the home and outside the home simultaneously. He calls for a reinstatement of the 'dignity of motherhood' in the traditional sense for those who choose to be mothers, while those women who choose careers, could be considered along with men as non-mothers.

Watanabe proposes this dichotomy of mothers and non-mothers to return the child's priority status in a mother's life while non-mothers will have as their priority a career.

It is evident throughout these papers, that the authors struggle to grasp the meaning for future generations of the present rapid changes in family structure and values. The imprint of technology exerts powerful forces, which, while improving life in some respects (e.g. decreasing infant mortality), endangers that which has been sustaining (e.g. support from an extended family). Mental health professionals would do well to attempt to reconcile the best of the technological as well as the traditional world.

ROBERT KRELL, M.D.

LEON EISENBERG, M.D. (U.S.A.)

THE SOCIAL CONTEXT OF HEALTH: EFFECTS OF TIME, PLACE AND PERSON

Health and illness can be understood only in a social context. The ways people live, the values they hold and the choices available to them are major determinants of 'perceived' health status as well as of 'actual' health status. It is not only that culture determines our views of who is well and who is sick but that the conditions of social life influence our very biology as well as our psychology. What we are, as well as what we think we are, is shaped by the way we live.

This year marks not only the Year of the Child but also the centenary of the birth of Albert Einstein. Permit me, therefore, to refer to the concept of relativity which proved so fruitful in deepening our understanding of the physical universe. In 1907, while Einstein was struggling to make the special theory of relativity, which applied only to systems moving with constant velocity, broad enough to accommodate accelerating systems, he had what he termed "the happiest thought of my life" (Einstein 1979).

> Just as is the case with the electric field produced by electro-magnetic induction, the gravitational field has only a relative existence. If one considers an observer in free fall, that is, from the roof of a house, there exists for him during his fall no gravitational field .... If the observer releases any objects, they will remain relative to him in a state of rest, or in a state of uniform motion .... The observer is justified in considering his state as one of 'rest'.
>
> The extraordinarily curious, empirical law that all bodies in the same gravitational field fall with the same acceleration receives once through this consideration a deep physical meaning. For, if there is even a single thing which falls differently into a gravitational field than do the others, the observer would discern by means of it that he is in a gravitational field, and that he is falling into it. But if such a thing does not exist – as experience has confirmed with great precision – the observer lacks any objective ground to consider himself as falling in a gravitational field. Rather, he has the right to consider his state as that of rest, and his surroundings (with respect to gravitation) as field free.
>
> ... The independence of acceleration in a free fall ... is therefore a mighty argument that the postulate of relativity is to be extended to coordinate systems that move nonuniformly relative to one another.

The relevance of this passage to our focus on health and illness is that, like Einstein's observer in free fall, we are equally blind to the effects of the 'cultural field' (akin to the gravitational field) on biobehavioral phenomena because we think and act within a cultural 'coordinate systems'. We only become aware of the field forces of our cultural system when we extend our vision to the study of other times, other places and other modes of social organization.

The definitions doctors employ for 'patient', 'disease', and 'medical care' are based upon a narrow biomedical perspective that ignores cultural relativity. To

S. H. Fine, R. Krell, and Tsung-yi Lin (Eds.), 'Today's Priorities in Mental Health' 35–48.

most physicians, patients are persons afflicted by disease or those who erroneously believe themselves to be so afflicted. From this standpoint, becoming well is a matter of being treated properly, if one is ill, or reassured accordingly, if one is not. The interesting questions, from this narrow medical viewpoint, concern the agents, the mechanisms and the treatments of diseases.

Far from being self-evident, this view underestimates the complexity of the transitions from personhood to patienthood and back. Community surveys regularly identify many more persons with symptoms and many more with abnormal physical and laboratory findings than the number who are under medical care (White, Williams, Greenberg 1961; Mechanic, Newton 1965). Are they simply unregistered patients in need of doctors, perhaps from lack of access or out of ignorance? Removing financial and geographic barriers *does* increase utilization but substantial numbers of 'non-patients' with symptoms and signs are found in populations covered by comprehensive health plans (Ingham and Miller 1976). If we invoke 'ignorance' as the cause, we take for granted that what doctors believe to be the right thing to do is correct and can be backed up by facts. But that is precisely what we need to determine.

In similar cases, becoming 'well' is not simply a matter of cure or remission of the disease process that made the person a patient. Every clinician is familar with the patient whose 'disease' has been treated successfully but who obstinately persists in complaining of symptoms, as well as with the one who insists on leaving treatment feeling 'well' when laboratory tests show active disease.

Underlying this conflict between the doctor and the patients is the difference between disease, as viewed by physicians, and illness, as experienced by patients (Eisenberg 1977). Modern Western physicians diagnose and treat diseases; that is, abnormalities in the structure and function of body organs and systems. Patients suffer illnesses; that is, unwanted experiences of changes in states of being and in the ability to fulfill social roles. Disease and illness do not stand in one-to-one relation. Similar degrees of organ pathology may generate quite different reports of pain and distress in different patients; illness may occur in the absence of disease, as witness the large number of visits to the doctor for complaints that do not have a discoverable biological basis. The course of disease is distinct from the trajectory of the accompanying illness (Twaddle 1977). It has been the triumph of modern medical sciences to learn very much more about disease than was known even a generation ago. In the course of that discovery, doctors' attention has been preempted by the virtuosity required to identify and treat disease, which has come to be regarded as the only 'reality'. Progress in the treatment of disease has been accompanied by neglect of the equally important task of treating illness. If we are able to attend to the patient as well as to his disordered biology, we must add to our understanding of diseases a correspondingly sophisticated understanding of illness (Eisenberg (1979).

Persons become patients when they conclude, almost always with the counsel of other family members, that they are ill, a judgement which is made against community standards of what it means to be 'well'. Thresholds for deciding that one is 'ill' vary with the person's very expectations of life. For poor people, pain and fatigue are often regarded as the way 'it's supposed to be'. Asked what it means to be sick, one respondent in a community study (Koos 1954) stated:

> Sometimes, I felt so bad I could curl up and die, but I had to go on because the kids had to be taken care of and besides, we didn't have the money to spend for a doctor. How could I be sick? How do you know when you're sick anyway? Some people can go to bed most any time with anything, but most of us can't be sick, even when we need to be.

Before a person becomes a patient by consulting a doctor, a whole series of transactions occur outside the official health care network and are never known to it. Community studies indicate that 75% to 90% of episodes self-identified as illness are managed entirely without recourse to the medical care system (Zola 1972; Hulka, Kupper and Cassell 1972). We know very little about how wisely families decide whether and when to consult a doctor. If only a tenth or a quarter of the self-diagnosed ill come to the doctor's office, is it the right tenth or quarter; that is, those who can benefit from medical care? We know the error rate is far from trivial, because we see many patients who fail to come until disease is far advanced as well as many who visit the office when they might have managed on their own. Medicine has barely begun to pay attention to the accumulating evidence that what doctors see in offices and hospitals is a grossly unrepresentative sample of sickness as it occurs in the community. When we examine a patient with symptoms suggesting localization to a particular anatomical structure, we assume we have found the source of the symptoms. We fail to consider the possibility that other individuals with similar structural abnormalities may be relatively or completely symptom-free. Yet such evidence abounds (Calin and Fries 1975).

If the biomedical aspects of practice suffer from insensitivity to the sampling problem, the consequences for the treatment of illness are even worse. The stubborn fact is that what doctors choose to call 'delay' in coming in for diagnosis is the *rule* in patient behavior rather than the exception (Twaddle 1977, Zola 1973). Most patients appear in the office with symptoms which have been present for weeks and months. Most people don't come in for most of their complaints most of the time; that's normal illness behavior. It is both useless and unjustly accusatory to ask the patient: "Why didn't you come in earlier?" when the important question is "Why did you come now?" The better we understand the triggers for deciding to see the doctor, the better we will be able to respond to the patient's needs (Mechanic and Volkart 1961). It is the patient who decides just how far to follow the treatment regimen after weighing its cost, estimating its usefulness, taking account of its impact on life style, and assessing its meaning to him. The doctor proposes; the patient disposes!

The beliefs, and thus the behaviors, of patient and physician move in trajectories guided by the 'gravity' of the cultural fields within which they live. Because those fields are ubiquitous, they are invisible. Laymen and professionals alike assume that 'diseases' are objective phenomena, independent of social constraints, when, in fact, the meaning given to the illness experience affects its course (Kleinman 1979). The most dramatic recent demonstration of the impact of culture on a mental disorder with a biological substrate is provided by the WHO nine nation study of schizophrenia (WHO 1979). Beginning with a cohort of patients diagnosed as schizophrenic by the application of common criteria, the investigators followed the course of their patients in each country for a five year period. Their outcomes proved to be remarkably different. Many more patients attained normal function in the developing than the developed countries, despite (or because of) the fact that so-called modern methods of care were far less available in the former than the latter. What accounts for the better outcome in developing countries? Is it the presence of the extended family with its multiple sources of social support for the patient? Is it differences between the social organization of traditional and modern societies? Or is it a difference in expectations conveyed to patients; namely, that recovery is to be expected when the disease is ascribed to spirit possession or that a chronic course is inevitable when the disease is viewed as a biological defect in the organism? Further research will be required to discriminate among the hypotheses. The point remains that what appears to be the same 'disease' follows a different course in different cultures (Waxler 1979).

The therapeutic encounter, whether with a Zambian shaman or a Western physician, involves the manipulation of symbols to give meaning to the illness experience and to place it within a frame of reference that is less frightening because it is more understandable. What we dismiss as the 'magical thinking' of a native healer is not as far removed from the beliefs of the modern physician as we tend to think. Both healer and doctor invoke the existence of invisible forces which 'explain' the chaos of disease (Horton 1967). Our patients, just as theirs, seek meaning; when we pronounce that the fever is due to a 'virus' (even when we lack the means to identify the virus or its products), both the patient and the doctor find the explanation comforting. The pronouncement, correct or not, makes the patient feel less ill because he is less worried; and it is likely to hasten the process of recovery by diminishing the physiological accompaniments of psychological distress.

The very biology of the human population is influenced by the nature of human society. Where human beings live, how many of them there are and the way they live has had profound effects on the evolution of the species and on the development of the individual. Measles and poliomyelitis did not become endemic in human communities until the agricultural revolution allowed enough people to live in one place to provide a reservoir for the virus to recycle itself (Black 1975). For some 500 generations of human history, such diseases exerted survival pressures on the species (Haldane 1956/7). Today we have vaccines which can sharply reduce and ultimately eliminate the incidence of new cases, as has been accomplished for smallpox. Yet measles continues to produce high death rates in African infants because of severe malnutrition and inadequate public health measures. Consider a second example of the intersect between social conditions and disease. The sickle cell gene, rare in other populations, has reached an equilibrium frequency of 10% in West African blacks because the heterozygote is resistant to falciparum malaria. Despite its cost to the homozygote, sickle cell disease persists as an adaptation to a malaria-infested environment. With malaria control, or with migration to malaria-free zones, the allele becomes entirely disadvantageous and its prevalence decreases (Cavalli-Sforza and Bodmer 1971).

Genotypic change continues into the modern era. Advances in medical care permit persons with genetic diseases to survive and reproduce. Because the diseases concerned are rare, the net effect on the human gene pool is slight. The most striking effect of industrial society, through improved living conditions and better medical care, has been to diminish natural selection pressures. Well over 95% of infants born alive in the developed world survive to the age of reproduction. The variance in the number of children born per woman does provide an opportunity for selection by differential fertility, but birth control is reducing that variance. If we ever do achieve a condition in which each couple simply has 2 children, there will be no room at all left for natural selection. Any subsequent evolutionary changes would be due to mutation and genetic drift.

Social change has had its greatest biologic effect on the phenotype rather than the genotype. In industrialized nations, there has been a secular decrease in the age of onset of puberty, which now occurs some 4 years earlier than it did a century ago. Although fertility begins later than menarche, because early cycles are anovulatory, there has been a comparable lowering of the potential age for conception. When to early puberty is added precocious adolescent sexual activity without the use of contraception, unwanted pregnancy is an inevitable side effect, an event which injures both infant and mother (Alan Guttmacher Institute 1976).

The higher morbidity and mortality for both mother and infant associated with adolescent pregnancy can be diminished by better medical care; nonetheless, there still remain detrimental social and developmental consequences for the immature mother and for the infant she is poorly prepared to nurture (Furstenberg 1976). In the U.S. in 1976, there were almost 800 000 pregnancies among unmarried women between ages 15 and 19. Had no contraception been in use, twice as many pregnancies would have resulted; had contraception been used regularly by all who did not want children, the number of pregnancies would have been reduced by half. Of the pregnancies that did occur, about one in 7 terminated in miscarriage and one in 4 in legal abortion. Punitive legislation in the United States to deny public funds for abortion will inevitably lead both to more unwanted births and to an increase in complications from septic illegal abortions (Institute of Medicine 1975). Public Health control measures must include: (a) sex education in the public schools, (b) the provision of contraceptives for those who are sexually active and (c) the availability of abortion for those who become pregnant and do not want children.

At the other end of the life cycle, there has been a steady increase in longevity.

There are now in the United States almost 25 million persons over 65; there will be 30 million by the turn of the century; there will be 50 million by the year 2030, even without further increase in longevity (Bureau of the Census 1976). The growing proportion of the elderly in the population is no purely American phenomenon; it characterizes all the developed countries. Were we to employ all of the effective health measures known to us, the proportion of the elderly would show further increase. Since the diseases of old age will continue to occur, the additional health costs incurred by the surviving elderly will more than offset the costs saved by early disease prevention (Gori and Richter 1978). This is not to argue against preventing or treating disease but to stress the urgency of social planning to anticipate the fiscal consequences of better health measures.

The new demographic profile of the industrialized nations, with increasing ratios of the elderly, has major monetary effects on retirement programs. In the United States, there were 16 workers for every beneficiary in the social security system in 1950. By the year 1978, the ratio had dropped to 3.8 : 1 and, by the year 2000, it will be 3.6 : 1 (Shabeloff 1978). The threatened bankruptcy of the Social Security Trust Fund was the moving force behind the recent decision of the U.S. Congress to raise the mandatory retirement age from 65 to 70. If postponing retirement diminishes the drain on pension funds, it brings other problems in its wake; unless the economy expands more rapidly than it has been, retaining the elderly in the work force must be at the expense of denying jobs to entry-level workers. Indeed, even without this change, major dislocations lie ahead. As a time-delayed consequence of the post-World War II baby boom, the number of potential workers in the 25 to 44 age bracket, 40 million in 1975, will grow to 60 million by 1990 (Flint 1978). Competition and strife in the workplace will mark the decades to come in the absence of appropriate social planning.

At its present birth rate, the U.S. will continue to increase in population until the year 2040 because of the large cohorts still within the fertile period. Events in Western Europe have outrun those in the U.S. In both France and West Germany, birth rates have fallen below replacement values and population decline has begun, with the expectable political consequence that agitation for pronatalist policies is becoming more marked (Kandell 1978). By the year 2000, the European continent will experience a population decline, four decades before the United States. The economic effects of the demographic reversal are already apparent. Over the past 50 years, social security contributions in Western Europe have jumped by 8% per year, about twice the annual economic growth rate. Whether national sanctions and incentives can smooth out the cycles of boom and bust in fertility rates remains an unanswered question (Parke 1979) but it has become abundantly clear that natal policy is a major issue for the developed as well as the underdeveloped world, which continues to be characterized by fertility rates that exceed gains in gross national product.

The increase in longevity for women, coupled with the decision to have fewer children, and the contraceptive technology to carry out that decision, has radically transformed women's lives. Two centuries ago, in much of the Western world, fewer than half the children a mother bore survived until age 10. With decreases in infant and child mortality, many fewer pregnancies became necessary to assure the same family size. Moreover, state pensions have diminished the reliance of elderly parents on the support of their children. At one and the same time, the demands of an industrial society foster the inclusion of women in the work force and working in turn influences decisions about preferred family size.

In the U.S. a social 'tipping point' has been reached. The majority of married women are now in the labor force (Eisenberg 1975). It is the woman who doesn't work rather than the one who does who feels it necessary to justify herself. It is a clear extension of human freedom that women can now attain a wider range of occupational roles. Community studies of the prevalence of depression in women indicate that the employed wife has fewer depressive symptoms than the housewife, though still more than men (Radloff 1975). Yet, as women have taken on social roles more like those of men, they have been acquiring male patterns of health-injurious behavior. Because more women now smoke, more will die of lung cancer, emphysema and heart disease. Deaths from violence may increase as well. Thus, women may lose some of their advantage in longevity. I do not cite these data as an argument that woman's place is in the home; to the contrary, I bring them forth as cautions against the adaptation of modal male patterns as the prototype for women. Both sexes would profit from a culture which made men more like women rather than the reverse (Eisenberg 1978).

An industrial society demands a mobile labor force. The consolidation of farming into agrobusiness diminishes the need for farm manpower. More and more of our population concentrate in metropolitan areas. Americans seem to be in perpetual motion. One in 5 families moves every year. On the one hand, this means fresh starts, less parochialism and more opportunities for young couples to begin their lives free of parental domination. On the other hand, it means loss of support from the extended family, fewer ties to the community and growing rootlessness and alienation. Urbanization, of course, is a world-wide phenomenon; its effects are more devastating in the developing world where barrios and favelas of grinding poverty surround cities whose population growth rate threatens their very survival (Turner 1977). People move because they despair of satisfaction where they are and they seek better education and more opportunity for their children elsewhere. The message is clear: without the investment of national resources to improve conditions in the countryside, migration will continue at the expense of both rural and urban areas.

In the course of these sociobiological transformations, the very nature of adolescence in the Western world has been radically altered (Eisenberg 1970). Its duration has been stretched at both ends of the age span. Puberty begins earlier and independent adulthood is attained later because of the longer period of formal education demanded by an industrial society. At the turn of this century, a bare 4% of American 18 year olds went to college; in the current year, half are enrolled in post-secondary education. If personal development were the prime motivation for college, the investment of time and effort might continue to be satisfying but the major thrust has been the hope of economic gain. Until recently, higher income did accompany a college degree; this is no longer so clearly the case (Freeman 1976). In Italy and France – and in India as well – university degrees are "fast becoming tickets to nowhere" according to the I.L.O. (Scully 1978). University students are in conflict. On the one hand, they protest the irrelevance of their education to their economic futures; on the other, they resist efforts to redirect the curriculum along vocational lines. Rising expectations conjoin with diminished opportunities to create a seedbed for political turmoil.

The problem is deeper than this. Western society behaves as though school is the only way for youth to come into adulthood. Schools have been viewed as the means to compensate for the inadequacies of family life, now that centrifugal forces pull the family apart and that the young spend increasing amounts of time outside the home. Yet the family such as it is remains a decisive influence. In a recent study from Warsaw, where the reconstruction of housing has diminished differences between neighborhoods, measures of cognitive ability in children continue to correlate strongly with the educational level of their parents (Firkowska, Ostrowska, Sokolowska *et al.* 1978). Socialization within the family remains crucial.

This does not mean that school is inconsequential. The point is that its benefits accrue differentially to those who arrive prepared for its academic demands. Professor Rutter's brilliant study of secondary schools in London (Rutter *et al.* 1979) has demonstrated that student outcomes are significantly influenced by the quality of the schools students attend, above and beyond differences in the characteristics of the children when they enter. Schooling did not wash out class differentials. However, behavior *and* attainment for both middle class and lower class children were far more satisfactory among those attending the better schools. Public education remains a crucial means of fostering human development.

We have tended to equate learning with what occurs in school. Yet, many failing students demonstrate mastery of a large array of social skills acquired outside the classroom. The separation of productive work from the family setting has sharply limited the day-to-day opportunities to learn vocational skills which, in traditional societies, are learned within the extended family. We in the West require a broader view of education than the schoolroom. Human development takes place over a lifetime and in every setting where people interact. Many young people can benefit from work opportunities interwoven with formal school sessions; in similar vein, adults should be entitled to 'sabbaticals' from work to return to the classroom. This is not a recipe for all; given the wide range of differences among individuals, varied mixes of learning and doing will be best suited for different persons. What is wrong is the present lock-step which demands the same sequence of schooling for all. For many, work and life experience can enhance the opportunity to profit from the classroom.

Changes in the school curriculum must go beyond opportunities for work-study. Lower birthrates mean small families; mobile families mean disrupted networks. Fewer of our children are given the responsibility to care for younger siblings and to learn about their needs. In view of the evidence for the powerful impact of parenting on child development, society must insure that those who will become parents are prepared for parenthood. Nursery schools and day care centers should be attached to secondary schools. Older students should be given the responsibility to share in the care of the young and should be taught the principles of child development. In one bold stroke, this will provide care for young children in an era when both parents work and will enable the parents of the future to learn what they need to know when they have children of their own.

If I have thus far stressed the relativistic effects of culture on human psychobiology, let me bring my paper to a close by stressing the one invariant in human nature. It's not new and it's not subtle. It can be stated simply: *people need people*. To love and to be loved, to belong to a human network and to feel that one matters to others are as vital to the preservation of health as air, food and water. This 'law' holds sway wherever human beings are found. It was as true in the past as it will be in the future. It is the basis of ethics *and* the precondition for mental and physical health. Let me highlight a few examples of the vast evidence for my assertion.

George Brown and his colleagues (Brown, Harris 1978) have studied the prevalence of depression among women in urban and rural settings in England. The most potent protective factor against depression proved to be an intimate and confiding relationship with a husband or a boyfriend; that is, a relationship in which feelings could be shared, whether or not there was sexual intimacy. In rural Scotland, those women least integrated into village life had the highest rates of depression. Miller and Ingham (Miller, Ingham 1976) sampled subjects from an Edinburgh general practice list. They found psychological and physical symptoms to be significantly lower among those who reported having friends and confidants. Henderson and colleagues (Henderson, Duncan-Junes, Byrne *et al.* 1978) studied a large, random sample of the general population of Canberra, Australia. They employed standardized interview schedules to assess levels of neurotic symptoms, extent of life stress and strength of social ties. It will not surprise you to learn that the greater the life stress, the higher the symptom score. What is more significant is that the more extensive the individual's social ties, the lower the symptom score. In the presence of stress, social ties provided significant protection against the likelihood of experiencing symptoms. The other side of the coin is represented by the large number of studies which have demonstrated an excess of mortality among widowed males and females during the several years after bereavement (Kraus, Lilienfeld 1959 and Young, Bernard, Wallis 1963)

The most impressive findings of all have recently been reported by Berkman and Symes (Berkman, Symes 1979) who studied the mortality experience of just under 5 000 men and women over a 9-year period. At the time of enrolment in the study population, each individual was asked about four sources of social contact: marriage; visits to and from close friends and relatives; frequency of attendance at church; and level of activity in group associations. When the four ratings were combined into a Social Network Index, the Index proved to be a powerful predictor of *life expectancy*. Death was more than twice as likely during the next nine years for those who were the most isolated in contrast to those who were the most connected. The Social Network Index was found to be associated not only with overall mortality but with four separate causes of death: heart disease, cancer, cerebrovascular disease and circulatory disease.

These findings are so startling that one is tempted to suppose that the causal chain is the other way around; namely, that those who died prematurely were isolated because they were already sick. But that was not the case. Health status at the start of the study was taken into account in evaluating the findings. Furthermore, it was not because the isolated drank more, smoked more or had poorer health practices, for these factors, too, were separately analyzed. The pathways by which social isolation increases mortality remain uncertain (Klerman, Izen 1977; Hamburg, Adams, and Brodie 1976) but the fact remains that strong social ties are essential for physical and mental health.

At the level of the individual doctor-patient relationship, it is this that accounts for many of the beneficial effects of the medical encounter. The doctor herself or himself is a valuable source of social support. The meaning the doctor gives to the illness experience by redefining it in terms of cultural metaphors reconstructs for the patient the relationship to self and others cast awry by illness. This is particularly evident in traditional societies where the shaman brings patient, family and community together in a healing ritual, such as the Navajo 'sing', which consolidates social relationships. These rituals have their counterparts in the West where illness provides the stimulus for relatives and friends to rally around the patient. In cases of chronic illness, the physician may suggest links to self-help groups. For some patients, behavior pathology is the cause of the social isolation. In such instances, social skills training and counselling may be helpful.

Yet, it is clear that individually oriented efforts to repair the damage after it has been done is an ineffectual and inefficient response to public health needs. Unless we attack disease at its source, social conditions will continue to generate patients much more rapidly than doctors can cure them. If there is to be any hope of maintaining health, prevention must become our major priority. To the extent that disease and illness result from social pathology (as I have argued repeatedly in this paper), is their prevention a 'political' or a 'medical' matter?

More than a century ago, Rudolf Virchow wrote: "Medicine is a social science and politics are nothing else than medicine on a large scale." As a member of a Medical Commission to investigate an epidemic of relapsing fever in Upper Silesia, Virchow concluded that its causes were more social than medical and insisted that "complete and unrestricted democracy" was essential to its cure

(Sigerist 1958). An advocate of free medical services for the poor, he insisted that medical care must be accompanied by social prophylaxis, including the right of each citizen to employment (Rosen 1958).

Radical critics of medicine belittle its effectiveness and implicate the structure of society as the source of most ills (Waitzkin 1974). Where Virchow had seen the medical profession as a part of the solution, the new critics disdain it as a part of the problem on the grounds that it serves to obscure the social roots of individual pathology (Navarro 1977).

Let us agree that there is little in the selection or training of the physician to suggest that doctors are reliable sources of wisdom or leadership for political reform. Yet, what doctors see, if their eyes are open, in the daily practice of medicine, enables them to identify the illness burden exacted by social injustice. Doctors have no greater wisdom than other citizens in devising remedies for that injustice. We do have an ethical imperative to call attention to its consequences.

If there is to be any hope of realizing the grand vision embodied in the Declaration of Alma Alta (International Conf. on Primary Health Care: Declaration of Alma Ata 1978), which calls for "the attainment of all peoples of the world by the year 2000 of a level of health that will permit them to lead a socially and economically productive life," that hope rests upon the commitment of each of us, professionals and nonprofessionals alike, citizens all, to the defense of the rights of man. Let me conclude as I began, by recalling the words of Albert Einstein (Einstein 1979):

> The existence and validity of human rights are not written in the stars. The ideals concerning the conduct of men toward each other and the desirable structure of the community have been conceived and taught by enlightened individuals in the course of history. Those ideals and convictions which resulted from historical experience, from the cravings for beauty and harmony, have been readily accepted in theory by man – and, at all times have been trampled upon by the same people under the pressure of their animal instincts. A large part of history is therefore replete with the struggle for those human rights, an eternal struggle in which final victory can never be won. But to tire in that struggle would mean the ruin of society.

Maude and Lillian Pressley Professor of Psychiatry
Harvard Medical School
Boston, Massachusetts,
U.S.A.

REFERENCES

Alan Guttmacher Institute
1976 11 Million Teenagers. New York: Planned Parenthood Federation of America.

Berkman, L. F. and Symes, S. L.
1979 Social networks, host resistance and mortality: a nine-year follow-up study of Alameda County residents. Amer. J. Epidem. 109:186–204.

Black, F. L.
1975 Infectious diseases in primitive societies. Science 187:515–518.

Brown, G. W. and Harris, T.
1978 Social Origins of Depression: A Study of Psychiatric Disorder in Women. New York: The Free Press.
Bureau of the Census
1976 Demographic aspects of ageing and the older population in the U.S. Curr. Pop. Rep.: Spec. Stud. Ser. P-23, #59.
Calin, A. and Fries, J. F.
1975 Striking prevalence of ankylosing spondylitis in "healthy" W27 positive males and females. New England J. Medicine 293:835–839.
Cavalli-Sforza, L. L. and Bodmer, W. F.
1971 The Genetics of Human Populations. San Francisco: W. H. Freeman and Co.
Einstein, A., *In* French, A.P., ed.
1979 Einstein: A Centenary Volume. Cambridge: Harvard University Press, 156–157.
Einstein, A., *In* French, A.P., ed.
1979 Einstein: A Centenary Volume. Cambridge: Harvard University Press. P. 305.
Eisenberg, L.
1979 Interfaces between medicine and psychiatry. Comp. Psychiatry 20:1–14.
Eisenberg, L.
1977 Disease and illness: distinctions between professional and popular ideas of sickness. Culture, Medicine and Psychiatry 1:9–23.
Eisenberg, L.
1978 La reparatition differentielle des troubles psychiatriques selon le sexes. Le Fait Feminin. Sullerot E. (ed.) Paris: Fayard. 313–331.
Eisenberg, L.
1975 Caring for children and working: dilemmas of contemporary motherhood. Pediatrics 56:24–28.
Eisenberg, L.
1970 Student unrest: sources and consequences. Science 167:1688–1692.
Firkowska, A., Ostrawska, A., Sokolowska, M. *et al.*
1978 Cognitive development and social policy. Science 200:1357–1362.
Flint, J.
1978 Oversupply of young workers expected to tighten job race. New York Times, June 25.
Freeman, R. B.
1976 The overeducated American. New York: Academic Press.
Furstenberg, F. F.
1976 The social consequences of teenage parenthood. Fam. Plan. Perspec. 8:148–164.
Gori, G. B. and Richter, B. J.
1978 Macroeconomics of disease prevention in the United States. Science 200:1124–1130.
Haldane, J. B. S.
1956/7 Natural selection in man. Acta Genet. Statist. Med. 6:321–332.
Hamburg, D. A., Adams, J. E., Brodie, H. K. H.
1976 Coping behaviour in stressful circumstances. Further Explorations in Social Psychiatry. Kaplan, B. H., Wilson, R. N. and Leighton, A. H. (eds.). New York: Basic Books, 158–175.
Henderson, S., Duncan-Junes, P., Byrne, D. G. *et al.*
1978 Social bonds, adversity and neurosis. Presented at the World Psychiatric Association Section Committee on Epidemiology and Community Psychiatry, Triennial Meeting. St. Louis, 18–20 October.
Horton, R.
1967 African traditional thought and Western science. Africa 37:50–71, 155–187.

Hulka, B., Kupper, L. L. and Cassell, J. C.
1972 Determinants of physician utilization. Medical Care 10:300–309.
Ingham, J, G. and Miller, P. McC.
1976 The concept of prevalence applied to psychiatric disorders and symptoms. Psychol. Med. 6:217–226.
Institute of Medicine
1975 Legalized Abortion and the Public Health. Washington, D. C.: National Academy of Sciences.
International Conference on Primary Health Care: The Declaration of Alma Ata.
1978 Lancet ii:1040–1041.
Kandell, J.
1978 Former French Premier seeks to spur lagging birth rate. New York Times, June 6.
Kleinman, A. M.
1979 Patients and Healers in the Context of Culture. Berkeley: University of California Press (in press).
Klerman, G. L. and Izen, J. E.
1977 The effects of bereavement and grief on physical health and well being. Adv. Psychosom. Med. 9:63–104.
Koos, E. L.
1954 The Health of Regionville. N.Y.: Columbia University Press.
Kraus, A. S., Lilienfeld, A. M.
1959 Some epidemiological aspects of the high mortality rate in the young widowed group. J. Chron. Dis. 10:207–217.
Mechanic, D. and Newton, M.
1965 Some problems in the analysis of morbidity data. J. Chronic Dis. 18:569–580.
Mechanic, D. and Volkart, E. H.
1961 Stress, illness behaviour and the sick role. Amer. Sociol. Rev. 26:51–58.
Miller, P. McC. and Ingham, J. C.
1976 Friends, confidants and symptoms. Social Psychiatry 11:51–58.
Navarro, V.
1977 Medicine Under Capitalism. London: Croom Helm.
Parke, R.
1979 Population changes that affect federal policy: some suggestions for research. Social Science Research Council Items 33:3–8.
Radloff, L.
1975 Sex differences in depression: the effects of occupation and marital status. Sex Roles 1:249–265.
Rosen, G.
1958 A History of Public Health. New York: MD Publications. 255–256.
Rutter, M. *et al.*
1979 Fifteen Thousand Hours. Cambridge: Harvard University Press.
Scully, M. G.
1978 Youth unemployment stirs international concerns. Chronicle of Higher Education, May 22.
Shabeloff, P.
1978 Life in a rose-covered cottage isn't rosy on $2,485 a year. New York Times, June 25.
Sigerist, H. E.
1958 The Great Doctors. New York: Doubleday, Anchor Books. 319–330.
Turner, F. C.
1977 La estampida Hacia las cuidades en Latino America. Inter Sciencia 2:31–41.

Twaddle, A.
1977 Sickness Behavior and the Sick Role. Boston: Schenkman-Hall.
Waitzkin, H. and Waterman, B.
1974 The Exploitation of Illness in Capitalist Society. Indianapolis: Bobbs-Merrill.
Waxler, N. E.
1979 Is outcome for schizophrenia better in nonindustrial societies? The case of Sri Lanka. J. Nerv. Ment. Dis. 167:144–158.
White, K. L., Williams, T. F., and Greenberg, B. G.
1961 The ecology of medical care. New England J. Medicine 265:885–892.
World Health Organization.
1979 Schizophrenia: An International Follow-Up Study. Sussex: John Wiley and Sons.
Young, M., Bernard, B. and Wallis, G.
1963 The mortality of widowers. Lancet ii:454–456.
Zola, I. K.
1973 Pathways to the doctor – from person to patient. Soc. Sci. and Med. 7:677–689.
Zola, I. K.
1972 Studying the decision to see the doctor. Advances in Psychosomatic Medicine. Lipowski, Z., (ed.) 8:216–236.

Dr. K. ZAKI HASAN (Pakistan)

CHILDREN AND FAMILIES IN THE THIRD WORLD: DILEMMA OR HOPE?

INTRODUCTION

The plight of children and families in the developing countries should arouse the conscience of the world for more than one reason. The whole question of man's survival on this planet has become linked with the problems arising out of poverty and deprivation on one hand, and of man's technical ability for self annihilation on the other. The extremely high infant mortality, the horrendous toll of infectious diseases and the abject poverty – with all its frightful consequences in physical deprivation, emotional instabilities, and social handicaps – are receiving growing recognition. Not so well appreciated is the fact that the historical process that created these societies of immense differences in wealth and social power has also made them extremely insecure. These societies are in a process of rapid change. The struggle for a new order gives rise to responses with a variety of normal and abnormal manifestations, with opposing forces locked in grim battle. The struggles raging in these societies (of the Third World) have a truly global character. One can only hope that the struggles do not turn into conflicts which produce either prolonged psycho-social disturbances or short-term intense aberrations capable of overshadowing the normal course of evolution of human societies. It is contended that the 'Dilemma' arises only when the compulsions of the inexorable process of change are not recognized, and the present is viewed in the framework of an unchangeable or slowly changing past. In other words, when the narrow interests of today blur the vision of a better tomorrow.

An attempt has to be made at developing a system of mental health care based on an understanding of the process of change. If at least the main aspects of psychosocial stresses of tomorrow can be predicted then indeed a more purposive mental health service can be delivered. True, that the manifestations of fundamental changes are bound to be as varied as they are complex. Paradoxes may abound but the time for a dispassionate reflection is now. Hope should replace the concept of dilemma.

As the tumultuous twentieth century draws to a close, it is appropriate to assess the conditions that children growing up in the year 2000 are likely to face. The extent to which trends in the prospective situation can be accurately identified and diagnosed will enable countries to take the firm steps needed to transform bleak prospects into brighter ones for nearly two billion children. The International Year of the Child has amply shown that there exists a reservoir of concern for children. Now is the time to reflect and to move firmly ahead.

S. H. Fine, R. Krell, and Tsung-yi Lin (Eds.), 'Today's Priorities in Mental Health' 49–58.

THE CURRENT SITUATION

There are 1.3 billion children under the age of 15 years in the world – about a third of the world's total population. Approximately 83% live in developing countries, where they form a high proportion (a recent estimate suggested 40%) of the total population. By contrast, not only do developed countries have smaller overall numbers of children but the proportion of children (approximately 25%) is also smaller.

There is also a sixfold difference in infant mortality rates. They range from one infant in six dying in Africa compared to approximately 1.1 per 100 in some industrial countries. Mortality rates in older children also vary according to the state of economic development. For example, the mortality rate in Mexico in 1972 for children in the age group range 1–4 years was 843 per 100 000 population compared to 79 per 100 000 in the Netherlands – a tenfold difference. In all countries the socio-economic level is the most important variable affecting mortality rates. Reliable morbidity data are difficult to come by, but it can be reasonably assumed that the main killers (infectious diseases and malnutrition) are also the main direct or indirect causes of morbidity. Reliable figures are, however, available for the proportion of people with food supplies adequate in protein and energy. It is a striking phenomenon that, while in the developed countries 3% of the population are below an acceptable lower limit for food intake, the average figure for developing countries is 25%.

Urbanization is proceeding rapidly, particularly in developing countries. Whereas 25 years ago a very small proportion of the population lived in big cities, it is predicted that by 1980 half the world's population will live in urban areas. Patterns of movement from rural areas to large cities vary, but in general the movement is motivated by the wish for better socio-economic conditions than what the rural life offers. Living conditions in large cities are highly unsatisfactory, and many city dwellers now live in large unhealthy shanty settlements on the edge of enormous urban conurbations with inadequate transport, housing, education, and health and welfare services. Migrant families have to cope not only with this poor material environment but with the lack of group support from close kin and friends, and from traditional cultural atmosphere.

Although figures are not readily available, it is likely that family breakdown in urban areas in developing countries is increasing. Certainly there are rising divorce rates in many developing countries. Increasing numbers of children are growing up in broken homes. Further, the illegitimate birth rate is rising in many developed and developing countries, and the children concerned (often born to very young mothers) are now, in some parts of the world, less commonly given up for adoption. Consequently, a larger number of children are being raised in single-parent families and therefore in a situation of social disadvantage. In developing countries the problem is made worse by the large number of children abandoned in city slums (World Health Organization 1977).

3. SOCIO-ECONOMIC STRESS

The physical, social and economic environment in which one lives, grows up and works affects one's health, susceptibility to illness and the chances of responding to an insufferable milieu by deviant patterns of behaviour.

The social environment is not readily subdivided as each aspect is dependent on the other; nevertheless the socio-economic status of a population is one element that can be usefully singled out because objective indicators are available by which it can be described and related to morbidity statistics.

Income and occupation, standards of housing, sanitation and nutrition level, provision of health, educational, recreational and other services may all be used individually as measures of socio-economic status and collectively as an index of the 'standard of living'.

There can be no doubt that in some developing countries economic progress and progress in preventative health programmes, better nutrition, improved sanitation and hygiene have been factors in reducing morbidity, increasing life expectancy, freeing people from an unremitting threat of ill health, and improving the quality of life. Nevertheless, poverty, with its accompaniments of disease and social disorder, remains a world wide blight.

Poverty causes illness by depriving man of his needs of shelter and adequate nutrition, and by exposing him to unsanitary conditions in which vector borne and other communicable diseases proliferate. This is evident not only in mortality figures for infectious diseases of the poorer classes, but also in their morbidity rates for cancer, arthritis and other chronic disorders, and in their high maternal and child morbidity rates.

The situation of the poor is further aggravated because in many countries they have less easy access to health services and often receive inferior care. Moreover, they are less well provided, with other services and amenities on which satisfaction and well-being depend, such as opportunities for leisure and recreation, security of work, and adequate schooling (illiteracy among the poor further shackles them to their underprivileged status).

Lastly, poverty debilitates its victims and predisposes them to what the developing world terms as fatigue and apathy, frustration and despair – the states of feeling that can induce not only psychological and bodily disease, but also crime, violence, and drug abuse. Indeed ecological studies of urban areas amply confirm that the rates of psychosomatic disorders, mental illness and alcoholism, are highest in areas of destitution and in the lower socio-economic classes.

But the phenomena of mental disorder in the poor are complex and not easily disentangled. The poor are subject to extreme stresses in their daily life which prevent their developing the defense mechanisms needed for a healthy mental life. They feel subject to oppression and injustice. Their social and cultural deprivation prevents them from undertaking joint organized efforts to bring about the required changes in the totality of their life pattern. Their violent individual protests are classed as criminal acts. The mentally retarded and the chronic mentally sick tend to fail socially and therefore drift into poverty. The standards of care available to them are usually totally inadequate.

There are grounds for supposing that effects on health depend on the context within which poverty is experienced, whether for example in an urban or a rural setting, and whether there are blatant contrasts between wealth and poverty. There are some ameliorating circumstances when poverty is in a rural community where a tradition of mutual support and camaraderie of shared adversity prevails (World Health Organization 1975). The child born into a slum may appear slightly better off than his rural brothers and sisters, but his poverty looms more acutely in the context of the unrealized potential inherent in the city's broader resource base. Relatively speaking then, the poor urban child experiences more deprivation than the poor rural child. For many, of course, the disadvantage is an absolute one as well (Hollnsteiner 1978).

4. URBANIZATION

There have been many studies of the general question of urbanization and economic development which have considerable significance. Of prime importance is the finding that rapid urbanization in many countries has out-stripped employment opportunities. This imbalance adds to the already enormous economic and social problems.

Asia and Latin America may be said to be over urbanized. In other words, people come to the city in large numbers not only because there is work in the factories, they come for other reasons as well, largely a push from the rural areas where the level of deprivation is higher than in the urban areas. Therefore, they have come to the city in the hope of bettering their circumstances. They may end disappointed but the change in their status is generally permanent and their place in the overall social struggle in the society changes.

The role of the cities in economic development has been a varied one. In the West the cities have been generative of great economic development and they are not parasites upon the rural countryside. In the developing countries, cities have been, and are, the hub of administrative and cultural activities. They have the economic power and the political clout. Their power over rural areas allows them to buy their products cheaply and sell them dearly to the city which enables them to live off the countryside. One of the phenomena visible all over is that the increase in trade of many cities of the developing countries being more related to the economic development of industrialized countries than to the economic development of their own country. In the West we find an integrated growth of the cities within a country, with various ones of them performing different functions, but in the developing countries often the cities provide no real support for the kind of economic development that we have in mind. At the same time these cities continue to show what we would call a modern pattern of consumption. People have been introduced to goods from the outside and have made them a part of their standard of living, but the standard does not come from the level of economic development in their own city but from the political power they enjoy.

It is therefore very important to plan for a balanced development of rural and urban areas. As far back as 1956 the Director General of ILO in his report said that:

> The cityward migration is typically unorganized and haphazard; the worker is unskilled; he has no experience of industrial work. Frequently he leaves his family behind in the village and retains close ties with them and a feeling of belonging to the land. There is a continual drifting back and forth between countryside and city by an unskilled unstable labour force which brings no lasting benefit to industry, to agriculture and to the worker himself.

Along with these problems of the male worker comes the problem of women or children who go with or follow their husbands and fathers to the city. There is child labour in the city. It is the cheapest labour available on the market. The pressure on the capitalist employer to reduce the cost of production by employing children is unrelenting. The pressure of poverty on the child to seek a job is also tremendous. The result is depressing, because many of the patterns seemed adequate in the rural setting when the children were working with their own parents on the farm but when transferred to the urban setting the child is much worse off. He works generally in the street trades, in domestic services, or in other trades which may well be harmful to his education and well-being. The child who was supervised by his extended family in the village finds himself without any such supervision.

The women workers, too, play a large role in the labour market in the city because their husbands cannot make a sufficient living for the family to subsist and their wages are lower than those of male workers. Oppressed on a double count, they are less militant and prove less formidable than men in industrial disputes. The nursing mother has to be absent to provide supplementary or even a primary source of income. This may find her spending a substantial proportion of her time away from home seriously affecting the breast feeding of the infant which compels early weaning. Substitute nourishment is never satisfactory at this critical period of brain development. Later, irregular meals, accidents, infected cuts, untended colds that soon develop complications and social deviations are common concomitants. Even if the mother takes one or more of the children with her to work it leads to other social problems.

Even under normal daily circumstances the house in which the child resides is often substandard accommodation. The house is frequently a shack where the child must suffer leaking roofs, where in winter the lack of clothing lowers his resistance to infections, and in summer the rains bring the large family into a small space which is also shared by dogs, goats, chickens and other animals. Unrelated families have to share the cramped space, a piece of cloth hanging between them providing the only symbolic privacy. That this is universal among the poor of the world is exemplified by the poignant description of the shacks that go for homes, by Lewis for the Martinez family in Mexico, (Lewis 1959) by Hasan for Pakistan,

(Hasan 1978) and for the African child by UNICEF (IYC-UNICEF 1979).

The tense emotional atmosphere that surrounds the child spring from multiple insecurities; economic, social and psychological handicaps which affect his family. For adults joblessness, or irregular or part-time employment, the need to work 12–16 hours a day take its toll on parents and by extension, on the child. Many a tired desperate father expresses his frustration through drinking and gambling. The fears and tensions engendered in the child by repeated quarrelling or actual violence between parents can have effects ranging anywhere from a neurotic personality to his running away from home. Unhappy adolescent boys and girls form a fertile ground for delinquency, vagrancy, drug abuse and prostitution.

Another source of strain on the family of the urban slum child is the ever-present threat of eviction. A government team may decide to turn land they are occupying into a harbour facility, a football stadium, or a bus depot. Soon after come the court notices and, in case of tenant resistance, bulldozers to demolish the houses and drive the occupants off the premises or forcibly relocate them. The process may take months or even years, keeping the anxiety level of the families high (Hollnsteiner 1978).

5. WOMEN AND DEVELOPMENT

In the process of social changes the weak and the oppressed have to bear the brunt of new forms of misery and deprivation. Women are the first line victims. Status of women worsens with migration. Her status in urban industrial societies has changed her role in the community. When left in the village she is worse off. But when in the city with her husband and not employed, her economic dependence is very often dehumanizing. Recent study of the role of women in societies which are changing from the traditional to the under-developed version of the modern society have brought to the fore many factors which go against the interest of women generally. A close study should make it apparent that the model of development which the countries have copied is one where the men are the main beneficiaries. This seems to have a negative impact on women's earning capacity as it does on internal structure of the family. Many aspects of this unfair development can be cited and one that deserves the most attention is the change in the pattern of cropping. From the traditional substantial crops there is a change to cash crops; this change is not only for the benefit of export but at the behest of governments whose main interest is to increase the prosperity of the land holding class. It has been shown in many countries that the so-called 'green revolution' has not been green but 'golden' only for the privileged few. The introduction of mechanized farming has replaced the women who used the scythe or the small knife. Their share of the harvesting operation is no longer available to them, and their family has to accumulate cash to buy the very product of the harvest at a much higher rate, a rate which is controlled by the market rather than by the simple system of barter which existed previously.

6. CHILD REARING

There is an extreme dearth of valid scientific data about the essential process of child rearing in the developing countries or evidence of the adequacy or otherwise of child rearing practices. One has, therefore, to depend on the scientific data that has been generated through research on the socially disadvantaged children in Western countries, especially North America. This may have valid implications for the developing countries and one can assume that malnutrition and other aspects of their poor socio-economic background have caused functional impairment in many children in these countries.

The rigid and oppressive social structure which exists in most developing countries must necessarily affect the institution of child rearing and education within that structure. Homes and school (from nursery to the University) cannot exist in the abstract. Within the structures of domination they function largely as agencies which prepare the individual for the existing society. The parent/child relationship in the home usually reflects the objective cultural condition of the surrounding social structure. If the conditions which penetrate the home are authoritarian, rigid and dominating, the home will increase the climate of oppression. The young people see the parent and teachers as authorities which are inimical to their freedom. Fromm has analyzed the condition which will create these situations; whether in the home where the child is exposed to a climate of indifference and oppression or of love and freedom; or in a socio-cultural context. Children reared in an atmosphere of lovelessness and oppression, who do not manage during their youth to take part in authentic rebellion, will either drift into total indifference, alienated from reality by the authorities and the myths the latter have used to shape them; or else engage in destructive action, which sometimes proves to be self-destructive (Fromm 1966).

The home atmosphere extends to the school where the students soon discover that in order to achieve some satisfaction they must adapt to the precepts which have been set from above. One of these precepts is not to think critically or to question the patterns, subjects or skills which their educators are attempting to impart to them, thus inclining them to concentrate on becoming a part of the power group and secure benefits which power can bestow. The students who go on to college and become professionals tend to repeat the rigid pattern in which they were reared. When they become part of the ruling group, or the group that advises the rulers, they continue to include in the planning process their objectives, convictions and preoccupations (Freire 1973). In fact they become alienated from the productive social functions.

7. EFFECTS ON PERSONALITY DEVELOPMENT

Interest in rapid cultural change in Asia and Africa has focused attention on the type of personality developed within an extended family with wide mutual interdependence, and within the small nuclear family which is increasingly characteristic of industrialized societies.

This has led the curious to look into the problems of personality development and socialization in those societies where a change in culture is taking place without appropriate movement in the sociological sense. The process of coping with a new culture requires the learning of new responses and skills, and the acquisition of new information. The process of coping with an unfamiliar cultural situation should be considered in relation to the major aspects of the process of adaptation.

Cultural adjustment requires the adequate functioning of personality in the changed environment. This presupposes that the change should carry within itself implied or explicit benefit. From the preceding discussion on urbanization it is clear that the benefit to the individual is not apparent, in fact the hardships are almost insurmountable.

The other major aspect is that of cultural competence which determines the capacity for acquiring new cultural knowledge and skills. The sociological change in the developing societies is a manifestation of discontent with their present status, and reflects their internal differences and contradictions. In most developing countries the pattern of relationships within the society are characterized by directness and immediacy of social relations. This makes less demand on the individual and he functions at a simpler level; but if the society were to undergo real progress there can be no doubt that the gap between the level of competence required and the level that obtains at the moment could be narrowed. Support for this optimistic view comes from the study by Taft on the immigrants to Australia (Taft 1966). He found that while education and secondary integration have a high correlation, primary integration is not dependent on education and general sophistication. Identity formation provides a concept within which self relization replaces adjustment. As a concept of maturation it is closely related to the phenomenon of change. But all this is not unequivocal. It has been shown that lower class children are able to profit from training (in learning to solve a concept problem) quite as well as middle class children with a mean IQ some 15 points higher (Osler and Scholrick 1968).

8. EFFECTS ON LARGE GROUP BEHAVIOUR

Although mankind divided itself into groups early in its history, claims to nationhood on lines prevalent in the contemporary world are a recent phenomenon. Economic domination, political subjugation, social backwardness, cultural handicaps and differences in religious beliefs or practices; any one or two or more of them are always the basis of claims for the right to exist as a separate sovereign and independent nation state. National struggles in Asia and Africa often transcend socio-economic and religious ideologies. The world of today stands divided against itself not only within the nations but also in the form of developed and developing countries.

The developing countries have between them 1700 million of the more than four billion inhabitants of this planet. They can be divided broadly into two groups. The larger and much more populous group consists of countries of Africa and South Asia most of which have achieved independence in the last 25 years. A much smaller group of countries have a small population but through the discovery of precious natural resources, mostly oil, they have become extremely prosperous in a very short time. On the surface the problems of these two groups of countries appear to be different; but this difference is more apparent than real. The social infrastructure that is necessary for a smooth evolution of a society and its progressive modernization does not exist in either group.

The key to a healthy change lies in the following:

A. Stratification that must eventually result should be of a type that is suited to the needs of the particular society. It should be so divided by occupation and income groups, and between agriculture and industrial bases of product location so that friction is minimized and each stratum complements the other.

B. The development and the change in attitudes during the rapid process of socio-economic development at both a group and individual level has to be achieved by a satisfaction giving participation of all the sections of the society.

C. This change should be indigenous to the area. The solutions evolved should be suited to the local conditions. The divisive foreign influences, languages, and alien models of social structure are to be avoided.

D. The socio-economic changes that occur rapidly instead of the evolution which has characterized the social development in the industrial countries, need to be the result of the political will of representative governments, as the most powerful social instrument. In the absence of a strong commitment to development policies, especially for the rural areas, the impact on the problems is not likely to be effective and broadly based.

E. There is an urgent need to develop social and educational institutions on a scientific basis which complement the socio-economic change. These institutions may be schools for the young in the rural areas, vocational centres for women, campaigns to expand functional literacy, societies for health education, child care centres for children of working mothers, training in skills for raising a family and operating a household, provision for facilities for recreation, etc.

F. It is imperative that the people should participate in the decisions regarding the priorities of development. Without a popular participation any of the social institutions mentioned will remain unused, and often misused; and unless they have indigenous roots they will not be able to perpetuate themselves.

G. To ensure success of any rapid socio-economic development the institutions which hinder development must be identified and removed. They may range from landlordism to monopolies or cartels along with their cultural, social, political and ideological counterparts.

In summary, only by considering the basic issues and doing something positive about them can nations of the Third World create a world of genuine options for the child's self expression and his contribution to humanity in the future.

Professor and Head,
Dept. of Neuropsychiatry,
Jinnah Post-Graduate Medical Centre,
Karachi, Pakistan.

REFERENCES

Freire, Paulo
1973 Pedagogy of the Oppressed. New York: The Seabury Press.
Fromm, E.
1966 In Socialist Humanism. New York. Quoted in Pedagogy of the Oppressed.
Hasan, M.
1978 Ramz-Zindagi (Urdu). Lahore: published M. Hasan, Temple Road.
Hollnsteiner, M. R.
1978 Basic Services for the Children of the Urban Poor in Developing Countries: a paper prepared for UNICEF.
Hollnsteiner, M. R.
1978 UNICEF Board Document.
IYC-UNICEF
1979 IYC Symposium Basic Working Document. Nairobi: UNICEF Regional Office.
Lewis, Oscar
1959 Five Families. New York: Basic Books, Inc. Publishers.
Osler, S. and Scholrick, E.
1968 Effects of Stimulus Differentiation and Inferential Experience on Concept Attainment in Disadvantaged Children. J. Exp. Child. Psychol.
Taft, R.
1966 From Stranger to Citizen. Tavistock, London.
World Health Organization
1975 Promoting Health in the Human Environment. WHO.
World Health Organization
1977 Child Mental Health and Psychosocial Development. WHO Technical Rep. Series 613.

MILTON H. MILLER, M.D. (U.S.A.)

THE TRADITIONAL FAMILY IN A CHANGING WORLD

Gore Vidal, American novelist, wrote, "I treasure most of all my old friends, the ones I have known for decades and have grown up with. They are like long novels. Having read this far, I want to see how it is all going to turn out."

I am steeped in family, and most of that is to the good. I am the father of three American, youth culture children now grown to their late twenties. Last week, I began my thirty-second year of marriage. My mother and father, both American born children of Austro-Hungarian Jewish immigrants have been married for fifty-four years. My father still practices law and gives me much unsolicited guidance. He and my mother are in regular touch with their three grandchildren, my children, one of whom will this week notify his grandparents that they will be great-grandparents soon after the start of the year 1980. We share my parents with my younger brother, Judge Stanley Miller of Indianapolis, his wife Mary and their four sons. My parents are strongly oriented around achievement, their own, their sons, their daughters-in-law, their grandsons (6), their grand-daughter (1), their grand-daughter-in-law (1) and soon, their great-grandchild, gender undetermined.

Each of my parents' parents – my grandparents – were married more than fifty years. All but one of them lived to see all of my three children. My grandfather, Mendel Miller, lived long enough to know that a baby was on the way and that the baby might well be named for him. It turned out to be Marcie, now 26, whose Hebrew name is Mindel, perpetuating the memory of the only grandparent who did not live to see her.

Along with my parents and grandparents, there were many other aunts, uncles, cousins. My Uncle Harry, known for his frugality and his suction kisses, gave me a quarter two or three times a year from the time I was about 14 till I was 32. I was to give a dime of that to my brother, Stanley. I had been named for Uncle Harry's father, Meyer Klein, so Uncle Harry favored me over Stanley. The only out and out black sheep in the family was my Uncle Jimmy, who drank and was married four times and who resembled another uncle, Uncle Jack, who was a Magistrate Judge, a non-drinker and straight arrow who was often embarassed when people mistook the two of them. My mother's only sister, Aunt Esther, who lived too few years, was a little silly sometimes and the weekly toys which she brought for my children, her grandnephews at the time, had a very short life-span. Most disastrous was a bubble-pipe hat with the soapy water stored in the top of the hat and a tube that came down to the pipe allowing a 3-year-old and a 5-year-old to make a grand entrance blowing bubbles – until the 3-year-old, nodded his head, got soapy water in his eyes and started to

S. H. Fine, R. Krell, and Tsung-yi Lin (Eds.), 'Today's Priorities in Mental Health' 59–67.

cry. Whereupon, the family in general and in chorus told Esther she was a fool.

I tell you all these things not only because I am also a fool, and nostalgic, but because that which I know with the greatest certainty is born of my own experience. The facts of life co-mingle with the eccentricity of family: winning is good, caring is essential, believing is logical, continuity is reassuring, living and obligation are synonymous and, last but not least, no suction kiss, no quarter.

In my own family and in many Western families, significant changes have taken place in recent decades. The nieces and nephews don't know each other. We are scattered in New York, Indiana, California and Canada. Where I once counted 'my family' as a group numbering sixty or more, we are now ten or twelve. That is large by contemporary standards.

At the same time, the events taking place in the contemporary family are the product of long developing changes in the way people think about themselves, their obligations and their hopes. I will be talking today about the matters of independence and interdependence, responsibility to self and responsibility to other purpose. In some respects, these very issues are rooted in the Renaissance.

In the field of sculpture, the Renaissance began abruptly in the year 1401 with the competition for the second bronze door of the Baptistry in Florence. It was open to 'skilled masters from all the lands of Italy'. Sculptors taking part were to depict a single scene, the Sacrifice of Isaac by the hand of his father, Abraham. The final competitors were Brunelleschi and the victor, Ghiberti, both of whose trial reliefs survive. The Ghiberti submission was the more traditional, medieval, a more mystical telling of the religious parable. The Brunelleschi version was phenomenological, depicting the anguish of the human figures and elevating the feelings and circumstances of the beings themselves to primary importance. Isaac and Abraham were not there to prove a biblical point. They were beings caught in an excruciating declaration of their personal life's meaning. The art historian, John Pope-Hennessy describes the respective entries and their significance in these words:

> The contrast. . . transpires most clearly in the central groups. Ghiberti's are ideal figures. The Abraham stands with a ritual knife in his right hand and the Isaac kneels resignedly upon the altar as he awaits the blow. With Brunelleschi, the figures are realistic; the Abraham moves forward with horror-struck expression, wrenching back Isaac's head and plunging the knife into his throat, and the face of Isaac is deformed by fear and pain. As we cross the frontier between these two conceptions, we enter the territory of Renaissance art. (Pope-Hennessy 1958)

As Brunelleschi had depicted the anguish and anxiety of the human situation, his friend and contemporary, Donatello, the greatest of Renaissance sculptors, depicted man in ultimate triumph. The statue of the young David with the Goliath head beneath his youthful foot was testament to the faith that man could climb to the top of the Cosmos. Brunelleschi and Donatello portrayed a cosmology whose strength and limitation is the history of the centuries that have followed. They elevated the hopes, the pride and the fears of the individual man.

Who is that individual? What is his purpose? What does he feel? What 'rights' does he have? What 'meaning' does he have? What of her?

Dr. Jules Masserman, distinguished psychiatrist and teacher, has written poignantly of the human circumstance discovered by the first people, pre-paleolithic men and women, graced with a capacity for boundless imagery and adaptive-integrative potential, yet faced with the stark realities of human existence, i.e. uncertainty, biological hungers, disease and penultimately, consciousness of the possibility of one's own death. For Masserman, the inevitable product of man's consciousness of finitude was the emergence of beliefs. The major beliefs are three; Masserman calls them the Primordial (Ur) Defenses and he sees them as universal. They are, first, our hope that we may somehow transcend this finite life and that there is meaning beyond ourselves. We call it 'Faith'. The second of the fundamental beliefs is that our work is important, that it matters, that the pictures we paint, the products we make and the stories we tell have a worth . . . and the same for mountains we climb, the diseases we cure and the noises from space for which we attentively listen. The third belief stems from the hope and joy we give to each other. It is a belief in love and the veracity of the peace which one discovers in holding hands (Masserman 1953).

A belief in transcendent spirit, a belief in the worth of work and a belief in love . . . these are the beliefs that sustain men and women worldwide . . . our cosmologies, however varied, are mostly variations on these three themes. Stripped of beliefs which seem as real as life itself, contemporary beings are in the same spot as pre-paleolithic ancestors, or perhaps we are worse off. The everyday urgency of finding food, protection and shelter was more diverting for people 40 000 years ago than it is today . . . . Although, as inflation progresses and the OPEC nations boost their prices, perhaps our own daily survival will become more uncertain, and thus diverting.

These three fundamental beliefs are intricately woven together worldwide in a wide range of fine weaves called civilization, tradition, religion, and national, personal and family values. We work because of faith and love. We have faith which causes us to work (for) those we love. Our love gives us faith and we work ceaselessly for both reasons.

As a psychiatrist these last thirty years, I find a restlessness in those who hold only two of the three basic beliefs; there is a profound imbalance in those who have come to hold but one of the beliefs. A belief in none is incompatible with life. Death comes equally to those stripped of belief by the depletions of disease and/or the demoralization of anomie.

My favorite story is about Wang Hwa, a Chinese man whose father had disappeared when he was a small child. Though he had grown to maturity and had married and had a son of his own, he still hungered and yearned for a father to whom he could be filial. With agreement of his own family, he found an old man whom he invited into his home for the purpose of receiving the family's filial attention. The old man was more than they bargained for. He drank, chased around and was generally demanding, but of course, the family honored its commitment. In the end, the story had a happy Chinese ending. The old man turned out to be Wang Hwa's long lost real father and he was also rich. The family was rewarded for their zeal. I often find myself photocopying the story to send to some 21-year-old student who comes up to me after one of my lectures to call me by my first name and complain that I don't know what I'm talking about, etc. In the story, Wang Hwa, carries out the customs that are traditional Chinese answers to the questions What is the meaning of life? How should life be lived? What is the relationship of my life to the order of the world? In a cosmological sense, 'Who am I?'

For the traditional Chinese, that cosmology is one which emphasizes inter-dependence and balance in all of life. One is oneself a part of unity of matter and spirit, a victim and master of human acts and the acts of nature. Things cannot be fine for me but bad for the universe; the sins of the fathers and greatgrandfathers and great-greatgrandfathers are all relevant and contemporary and influential in determining one's well being. They are all there. It is all there in a closed universe where nothing is irrelevant or time limited. 'Filial piety' is not simply good manners born of careful upbringing. Ancestors honored and well cared for the natural allies to fight off, balance, and/or neutralize those omnipresent forces which, all know, pervade this universe and bring disappointment and ill to each of us. In turn, my actions, misdeeds, omissions or derelictions harm not only me but the universal balance. A good Chinese friend, living in the United States, was explaining why divorce was not possible for her though her problems with her husband were considerable. She explained that there is no divorce in her lineage and that if she were to divorce her husband their children would be seriously handicapped in finding mates. Other families with children who would be potential husbands and wives for her children would be fearful that a disruptive element would constantly be present in that lineage, a restlessness of ancestors that would bode ill in the future of the couple. Nor did my friend feel that she could seek refuge in divorce after all her children were married. There was the matter of the success of her children, their health, the health of grandchildren and the marriageability of those grandchildren. No, for her, life is responsibility. One accepts inter-dependence, not independence. One is linked forever in a network of beliefs and obligations. Obedience is a virtue.

It has come to pass that obedience to a network of hierarchically determined beliefs and obligations is no longer seen as an obvious virtue in many Western homes. Brutality and world catastrophe have been perpetrated in the name of filial piety, patriotism and obedience to father or fatherland. While I hunger at times for the comforting familiar boundaries imposed by narrow loyalties, I'm quite sure that in our world of atomically armed nations there will be no hope for survival without a change from the values and cosmologies inflexibly held in the first half of the 20th Century. Basically, those cosmologies were handed from parents, through children to grandchildren. A main emphasis was on being a 'good child' whether one was 6 or 60. Loyalties were to 'one's own' with the first obligation hierarchial, to the father–grandfather. Older peoples 'rights' and requisites were perpetuated along with the 'traditional values'. That system had obvious ecological strengths, particularly in rural societies living in danger of scarcity or external enemies. I have summarized that traditional structure in the following allegory:

THE BEGINNING OF CIVILIZATION

While handwriting as we know it had yet to be invented, for Ajote – who was now thirty-eight – it was unmistakeably on the wall. He slept uneasily in his cave, feeling closed in, surrounded, trapped. In the early morning hours, he often thought of the afternoon some thirteen summers before when he had stealthfully slain the headman of the tribe in which he lived. A few discreet weeks after the murder, he had taken the cave of the the headman and with it leadership of the group. He ruled during the succeeding thirteen years. But now, Ajote began to cough and to spit red which was a certain beginning of a loss of strength and power. For a headman, such loss meant death. Ajote, frightened, had attempted to do a little political friend-making, trying to warm up to some of the younger men by making friendly gestures on the hunts. But, as is usually the case with appeasing gestures motivated by fear, these efforts made him only more afraid.

He thought of fleeing, but to where? The extent of his world was only the hunting area of the tribe – the caves in which they lived, the lake below and some fifty square miles of forest bounded by the far hills. He was restrained from penetrating those boundaries, recalling the murderous treatment he had afforded a strange man who had fled from those far hills and come toward their lake three summers before. His apprehensiveness mounted as he recalled that the murdered stranger had been, like himself, an older man. Why had he come?

One day, while Ajote was coughing and spitting he saw the most agile and unfriendly of the younger men watching him. He felt he had no hope and decided to flee from the group. That night, while the others slept, he left the cave, carrying food and a weapon. He reached the far hills at dawn and an hour later lay hidden one hundred yards from the central gathering place of the tribe who lived beyond the hills. Several of the young men in this group resembled the older man who had been slain. Ajote experienced great fear and decided to return to his own tribe. However, he took four days to make that five-hour journey and when he returned he had carefully practiced this story which he told with great feeling to the people of his tribe: A dream had foretold imminent danger to the group. He had seen an image of many of their women and young people killed. He remembered specifically the crushed head of the strong young man who had observed him coughing. In the dream, a strange beast, half-mortal, half-animal, had led him, Ajote, to the far hills to avenge the slayings. On awakening he had immediately gone to the far hills as instructed and discovered that the people there were making preparations for an attack as had been predicted in the dream.

The events that followed made Ajote the leader of the group as never before.

He had foretold the grave danger. He had caused his tribe to send its younger men over the hills in time to head off the assault. In that war, the strong young man who had observed Ajote's coughing was, as foretold in the dream, killed. Ajote subsequently made known to all what was necessary to preserve the group against other enemies. All the other young men were very respectful to Ajote. This was the beginning of once-upon-a-time civilization . . . .

In the last thirty years in North America, as you all know, we have been witness to remarkable changes in social structure and values. The struggle of Brunelleschi to individuate mankind as unique in a Godly world has reached a point in our time when many individuals feel that they have been individuated from mankind as well. Many factors are responsible; most important, I think, are the impact of television and the demise of most extended families with urbanization. The first generation to grow up with television in the United States is now approaching thirty. They were the first human beings in the history of the world whose education was not specifically supervised and controlled by the parents and/or leaders of the village and community. This is a change of overwhelming importance. Urie Bronfenbrenner estimates that:

> American children under six spend an average 50 hours a week watching television. By the time the average American youngster graduates from high school, he or she has spent more hours watching TV than any other activity except sleeping.

He believes that parents are replaced in the lives of most children by TV, peers and loneliness and that the consequence is a society which is temporarily off balance. He writes:

> What matters most for many people is their own growth and happiness, their own self-fulfillment. We seem to be sunk in individualism. We want so much to 'make it' for ourselves that we have almost stopped being a caring society that cares for others. We seem to be hesitant about making a commitment to anyone or anything, including our own flesh and blood. To be sure, individualism has helped bring about extraordinary solo efforts by many Americans. But we have entered a period of history when we need to put other, neglected values on the scale too. (Bronfenbrenner 1977)

The second major change is in family structure with a loss of extended family patterns and the emergence of a learning and teaching of values from and by other young people. When I was growing up, I was outnumbered by parents, grandparents, aunts, older cousins, teachers. It was 30 adults impinging their ideas and demands on me. Twenty years later, it seemed to me that my wife and I were outnumbered by our children's friends twenty to two. Perhaps I sound paranoid, but I know that raising young people when the kids outnumber the adults can be rather difficult.

I'm going to be citing some statistics pointing to the magnitude of social change in my country. But I think we need to look at these findings in perspective. The main truth about people is that they have struggled with vast problems through the millenia, and then, after a while, some new humans and new problems emerge and with them, new solutions.

In the United States of America, to which I have returned after 6½ years in Canada, the pendulum has swung far to the side of independence rather than interdependence and single parent families rather than extended families.

1. Forty percent of American marriages end in divorce. In California, in March of 1978, there were 13 000 divorces and 10 000 marriages. Nationally, that month, there were 150 000 marriages, 100 000 divorces. In 17 years, the rate of divorce has tripled. The census bureau revealed the other day that more than 20% of families are single parent units, mostly mother and children. There are probably three times as many single parent families as there are 'typical families' with father working and mother at home with a couple of kids. Presently, there are eight times as many couples living together without children as there are units with father working and mother and kids at home. The one earner family is a minority in the United States.

2. There are significant changes in attitudes concerning the responsibilities between parental and children's generations. The eschewing of responsibility for parents is finding a parallel in attitudes of parents with regard to their children. The commitment, 'I would do anything for my children' is losing force. Pollster Daniel Yankelovich finds that some 40% of American families with two parents and one or more children under 13 years of age belong to a 'New Breed' which is committed to duty to self(ves) over duty to others, children included. He contrasts these parents with the more traditional American value which declared, 'I work for my children. My reward is their success (and appreciation)'. The New Breed says instead, 'There is a clear limit to what we will sacrifice for you. We have our own lives to lead. And when you are grown, in turn, you owe us nothing'. This attitude correlates with various marital satisfaction studies which show a precipitous decline after the birth of the first child and a rapid improvement after the last child has left home. Still, the hope of finding 'it' with her, or him, is very strong in the United States. Ninety percent of our people marry, and of those who divorce, 80% remarry, mostly within the first three years after their divorce decree.

In a way, the most dramatic aspect of the INDEPENDENCE tendencies in the last decades is the INDEPENDENCE OF THE GENERATIONS. The first generation in the pattern moved out from an intense sense of responsibility for their parents. Their children and grandchildren in turn have been freer to divorce, not only the first spouse, but the children as well. But that much independence is not much fun and a new pattern of the remarried or childless couple whose cathexis and commitment is within their own generation is more prominent in the United States. Change of such a magnitude touches many lives and for some the consequences are sad indeed. Suicide is the leading cause of death among young people. The majority of young people, cast on their own, tumble but land on their feet. A certain group are stark casualties of an independence with which they cannot cope. My wife and I came to know well a large number of our children's contemporaries and I must say that many of the drop outs of the 1960s are still out and sadly so. I am certain that our own children would be doing much less well than they are if they had not received sustaining and sometimes intense doses of parental and grandparental support (encouragement, and much more). I think that hasn't changed much. To have an advantage – – – is an advantage. Although we know in an intuitive way that the children of divorce pay a price, there has been relatively little study of them. Judy Wallerstein and Joan Kelly in San Francisco have followed several groups of children of divorce for some ten years. Their results show that there is much variation, but a large percentage, a quarter and more, show significant deterioration of psychological adjustment of the children in the first year of divorce. They point out that it is not simply the act of divorce which is important, but the chain of events that are associated and additive in aggravating the child's situation. Particularly important are the problems and mood of the mother and her adaptation to life as a divorced woman. (Kelly and Wallerstein 1976). Each year in the United States, a million mothers, a million children and a million fathers are participants in the divorce process. One's hope for each is that their personal beliefs are strong and resilient and that they are among friends – if not family. We've not yet found the way, in Western society, to safeguard the children whose well-being depends upon the well-being of a single adult. This is a very serious problem in an era of great mobility and general social change. In the State where I live, California, it is a crime to fail to report acts of violence upon children and we are seriously attempting to take leadership in declaring that the child lives with a family but belongs to the future.

In my own work as a psychiatrist I find that my interests and efforts are increasingly turned toward supporting those social endeavors which I feel elevate and strengthen the belief systems of people. I believe in self government, physical recreation, friends, shared undertaking, women in highest offices, couple-family therapy, couple vacations, hopes. I have come to feel that, while we therapists greatly help people, it is through their loving relationships that they find full cure. Love cures them. I am mystified by this period in history – and I think it will be time-limited – when allegiances are so brief. I am mystified because almost everybody I know tells me that life is at its best with the people you love.

Deputy Director,
Mental Health Department, Los Angeles County.
Professor and Chairman,
Department of Psychiatry,
Harbor-UCLA Medical Center,
Los Angeles,
California, U. S. A.

REFERENCES

Pope-Hennessy, J.
1958 Italian Renaissance Sculpture. New York: Phaidon Publishers Inc. p. 2.

Bronfenbrenner, U.
1977 The Disturbing Changes in the American Family in *The American Family*. Feb. 23–26.

Kelly, J. B. and Wallerstein, J. S.
1976 The Effects of Parental Divorce: Experiences of the Child in Early Latency. American J. Orthopsychiatry 46(1), pp. 20–32.

Masserman, J. H.
1953 Faith and Delusion in Psychotherapy. American J. Psychiatry 110:324–333.

SHOICHI WATANABE (Japan)

THE NEW DICHOTOMY OF MANKIND: MOTHERS AND NON-MOTHERS

It is evident that we are living in a schizophrenic world. A few years ago the whole world celebrated the International Year of the Woman. The main theme of that international congress was how to liberate women from their families. On that occasion the family was almost regarded as the root of all evils. This year the whole world is celebrating the International Year of the Child. The main theme is of course how to make children happy in their respective families, and the family is being recognized as the root of happy children again.

In former days we used to think that women and children are happiest in their families together. Now, children are more often than not the enemies of those women who have been liberated or will liberate themselves. Women are grown-ups and children are small and helpless. The consequences are evident. Women are getting the upper hand of children everywhere, and children are losing ground everywhere. However, children can and will revenge themselves for the wrong they have suffered by becoming juvenile delinquents or neurotics, or staying mentally retarded. Such being the essence of the matter, the problem of the worldwide dilemmas of children and families needs to be considered in connection with women's liberation.

Human beings have been accustomed to the predominant dichotomy – the dichotomy of man and woman – for a very long time. It has been assumed by monotheistic believers that this dichotomy of human beings is God's will. *Fiat voluntas tua*! In the Western World the ideal image of happy woman has been a mother staying at home with her children. On the other hand those agnostics and atheists who do not believe in the story of Genesis have no alternative but to accept evolution. According to this theory mankind has come to have two sexes as a result of hundreds of millions of years of evolutionary development, and female anatomy convinces us very easily that women are evolutionally predetermined to gestation, parturition and lactation. This means simply that women and children are inseparable. Either from the fundamentalist point of view or from the evolutionary point of view a family where a mother and children live together seems to be the most natural unit of human existence.

It follows from this conclusion that the women's liberation movement is perhaps a modern type of heresy of an egregiously unnatural, unscientific movement, though we sense that there is something pathetically true about the assertions of women's libbers. Orthodoxy has maintained that every heresy contains a small particle of truth, though not the whole truth. At any rate, the women libbers' disdain of the family cannot be explained simply as a particle

S. H. Fine, R. Krell, and Tsung-yi Lin (Eds.), 'Today's Priorities in Mental Health' 69–72.

of truth, because their movement is flatly against the traditional idea of a happy family where a mother is devoted to the care of her children.

During the last war my sisters used to congratulate themselves on having been born women, because they were exempted from being drafted into the army. It was my mother's lifelong sincerest wish to become a woman who could afford to remain at home and devote the prime part of her time and energy to her own family and children. Owing to a series of misfortunes, however, she was obliged to work outside the family for most of her life. She was an able woman and was trusted everywhere. In a word, she was tolerably successful in the world. I know very well that she regretted having been obliged to work outside the family. My sisters' predominant wish was to become women who could afford to stay at home and devote their time and energy to their own families and children. I assume it was also the case with most women in the Western World. By contrast, nowadays many married women and even young mothers feel themselves inadequate unless they are working outside their families and earning money. Why have women become so eager to work outside their own families, entrusting their helpless children to other people's care?

It seems to me that there are two main reasons for this phenomenon. One is the ideological influence of Marx-Leninism, and the other is the tremendous development of technology.

First of all, let us have a glimpse at the Marx-Leninist idea of the family. From the very beginning Marxist leaders were of the opinion that a woman in the family is one of her husband's possessions and that a woman working in the family is a form of private property just like a cow or sow. Vladimir Ilich Lenin maintained that women should be liberated from work in their families and be made to work in factories or offices. Lenin and his followers regarded the family as the bastion of egoistic individualism. They have been intentionally trying to disintegrate the traditional idea of the family. From this perspective of society the Soviet Union may well be called the most advanced country in the world. In this connection it should be pointed out that most women's libbers in Japan are leftists. They want to have lots of public nursing institutions so that mothers may work outside their families, and thereby be separated from their children for most of the day.

In this socialistic effort to disintegrate the traditional family it is easy to discern that working for the state is for women's libbers more important than working for their own children. The state is first priority and family life is not held in high esteem. Thus, about 80% of Russian women of workable age are employed outside their families, a figure comparable to that of Japanese men of working age. Both men and women are to work outside their families. Their children are to be brought up and taken care of by the state. Children belong primarily to the state, not to their parents.

This is roughly the Marx-Leninist view of families and children, and we know it has often been regarded as a most progressive idea by a considerable number of Western intellectuals.

Secondly, let us have a glimpse at the influence of modern technology on the family. The rapid development of technology has greatly changed the nature of work both outside and inside the family. Labor outside the family used to be more cruel and more muscle-oriented than today. Just imagine how physically excruciating it must have been to ride a horse through woods and muddy fields for weeks on end. But it was the job of cavalrymen. And imagine too how physically excruciating it must have been to work for ten hours a day six days a week in a primitive iron foundry. Very few women could have been eager to work side by side with muscular men under such conditions. Today the muscular parts of all jobs have been replaced by machines and gadgets. Just think of a fork-lift. Work conditions have improved at an astonishing rate. My sisters would have shuddered at the idea of becoming officers in the old Japanese army, but their daughters are regarding commissions to the present Japanese army as offering them an attractive career.

Within the family the mother used to be its focus. In agricultural areas the mother not only prepared meals but also made cheese, butter and sausages. Even in towns it was a tremendous amount of work to keep house and bring up children without the help of electric gadgets. Without an able and devoted mother a family could not possibly go on living. Nowadays, there are automatic washing machines with dryers, huge refrigerators, powerful vacuum cleaners, efficient dish washers and unbelievable microwave cooking ovens. Anyone can keep house, even a man. How miraculous!

As a result, women have lost their prestige and identity, or *raison d'être* within their families. They now feel obliged to prove themselves in other ways. The same technological development that has made women feel unimportant inside their families has made the jobs outside their families more congenial and much less excruciating than they used to be. It is only natural that more and more women should get out of their families to prove themselves by earning money.

In former days the male role and female role in the family and society were distinctly different and were regarded as complementary to each other. If the father was compared to heaven, the mother was compared to earth. Nowadays, earth wants to be heaven, and there are two heavens and no earth in increasingly more families. I am very well aware that girls can be as bright, as brainy, as ambitious as boys. I am very well aware that women can work as well as men in most fields. In short, we can almost ignore the differences between man and woman. In this sense the assertions of women's libbers are right. Marx-Leninism and modern technology have been unsuccessful in abolishing the antediluvian dichotomy of mankind into man and woman. Now, a woman can become not only a queen but also a prime minister.

For all this, however, one solemn fact does remain: only women can become mothers. Only women can perform such vital functions as gestation, parturition and lactation. This is God's will, if we believe in God. This is the inevitable result of evolution, if we believe in science. There is no escape from this unalterable fact. Even the most extreme Marx-Leninist, even the most extreme women's libber must admit this. There is one escape from this destiny, that is for the woman to remain childless. We know many respectable career women who have given up the idea of having their own families or children for the sake of their careers. But most women are not so resolute. They want to have both career and children. This is a very dangerous situation for such women are often inclined to feel ambivalent. They want to have the experience of being mothers, while at the same time they want to get free from their own children as soon as possible. Is this not an atypical psychological attitude which leads towards a necessary evil? Children in the modern world are not the pride of women, but their necessary evils. Mothers today seem to have lost the genuine and unmitigated joy, the sense of personal fulfilment that their mothers used to have. Most children feel it instinctively if their mothers prefer their own jobs to them, or if their mothers regard them ambivalently. This is hardly a wholesome atmosphere for children. Common sense tells us that children need to feel their mothers love them more than anything else in the world.

I remember standing at the doorway and seeing my mother off to work. I did not think even for a single moment that my mother loved her work more than me. Though I was an infant, I instinctively understood that my mother was forced to go to work even though she wished to stay at home. On the contrary, many children today seem to have lost confidence in their mothers' love. Suppose I were an infant now and had to choose between a mother who was a beggar and a mother who was an executive in a big business. If I were to choose the former, I should have to go around begging for food hand in hand with my mother. Were I to choose the latter, I should have to be sent to a nursing house where somebody else would take care of me for most of the daytime. If I were to be compelled to choose between these two kinds of mothers I would not hesitate to choose being a beggar's son. A beggar's son can eventually become affluent in the future and will have a very sweet memory of his togetherness with his loving mother. On the contrary, the female executive's son will not appreciate his childhood very much. His memory will tell him that he was inferior in importance to his mother's job. He may well tend to be spiritless, lethargic and devoid of ambition, because he knows ambition for a career was his mortal enemy, or he may become violent and antisocial. It is sometimes suggested that the quality of the emerging generation seems doomed to deteriorate. To stop this deterioration, we must reinstate the dignity of motherhood. As the women's libbers say, the traditional dichotomy of mankind into man and woman may have ceased to be as valid as it used to be. So I should like to suggest a new kind of dichotomy of mankind into mothers and non-mothers. Non-mothers may and should work as much and as hard as they wish in whichever way they like. But mothers should, in principle, stay at home with their children as exclusively as possible while their children are young. Only this new dichotomy will enable our future generations to be happy.

Professor of English,
Sophia University
Tokyo, Japan

SECTION THREE

CHILDREN'S RIGHTS

INTRODUCTION

In the Year of the Child, children's rights should be a paramount consideration. Prof. Rae-Grant emphasizes that legislation is often not only useless in protecting children's rights, but can also cause impediments to such rights. He cites two examples: the Juvenile Court Act of Canada allows juveniles a less formal court setting but denies them the rights to cross-examine, to confront hostile witnesses and to avoid self-incrimination. In addition, a child or adolescent admitted to a residential mental health centre may not appeal and has little say about his disposition after leaving this centre.

He traces the history of the rights of children from Greek and Roman times to the present. Ms. Robbins also traces the history of these rights with speical reference to the role of the adult volunteers in the mental health associations. These associations can act as effective guardians of children's rights and can lobby for implementing them in legislation and in day-to-day practice.

Dr. Ehrhardt shows how the Universal Declaration of Human Rights adopted by the United Nations in 1948 also includes children, and that the family, although protected from interference by the State, must allow the children and juveniles opportunities for survival and growth. If these are not provided, the State intervenes. These rights suggested by the United Nations have formed the framework for laws in several countries.

All the authors stress the importance of maintaining not only the physical health of children but also their emotional health. Thus children have a right to obtain mental health services.

Each author tackles the question of children's rights from a different perspective – Professor Rae-Grant historically, Ms. Robbins from the Mental Health Association volunteer viewpoint, and Professor Ehrhardt by reviewing the international legal scene. Some practical suggestions for implementing these rights are made.

STUART FINE, M. B.

S. H. Fine, R. Krell, and Tsung-yi Lin (Eds.), 'Today's Priorities in Mental Health' 75.

Prof. HELMUT E. EHRHARDT, Dr.med., Dr.phil., Dr.jur.h.c. (West Germany)

HUMAN RIGHTS AND THE RIGHTS OF THE CHILD

It was in 1902, in a book which was read all over the world, that the Swedish educator Ellen Key proclaimed the 'century of the child'. If we ask ourselves now, in the last quarter of this century and during the 'Year of the Child', what has actually become of this proclamation, we have to recognize that the outcome has been quite different from what one could foresee at the turn of the century. The rapid and sweeping changes in the social structure of the industrial nations resulting from the frantic pace of technological progress confronted the societies in these countries with a wealth of problems. They were unlike any they had previously encountered, particularly those involving the younger generation, the children and adolescents. The effects of two world wars have fundamentally changed our view of the universe. We have almost become accustomed to think and to live in terms of global antitheses such as east and west, north and south, rich and poor. Traditional values are constantly questioned or have already lost their validity, although we are still without a hint as to the nature of those values which must replace the old. The problems of the developing nations present a world-wide challenge and an obligation unknown to former generations.

THE UNITED NATIONS AND HUMAN RIGHTS

The United Nations Organization, despite all its weaknesses and shortcomings and the criticism voiced of it, continues to reflect the most important attempt since the Second World War to establish a new value system on a world-wide scale. The motivation of the fifty participating nations which signed the *United Nations Charta* in June, 1945 at the San Francisco Conference was doubtless quite varied and not only idealistic. This, however, had no bearing on the substance of the Charta or the fact that it entered into force on October 24, 1945, United Nations Day.

The United Nations derives its mandate to promote human rights from Article 55(c) of the Charta. This states that it is necessary in the interests of friendly cooperation between the nations to promote "universal respect for, and observance of, human rights and fundamental freedoms for all without distinction as to race, sex, language and religion".

According to Article 2, Paragraph 7 of the Charta, the United Nations shall not "intervene in matters which are essentially within the domestic jurisdiction of any state." This *principle of sovereignty* is characteristic for the limitation of the effectiveness of the United Nations, which is after all not a world government.

S. H. Fine, R. Krell, and Tsung-yi Lin (Eds.), 'Today's Priorities in Mental Health', 77–83.

The body within the United Nations which is charged with the promotion of human rights is the Commission on Human Rights, established by the Economic and Social Council. The Commission consists of representatives of 32 United Nations member states. The geographical distribution of the Commission members and the rules of procedure demonstrate that usually questions of the protection of human rights are essentially political questions, the resolution of which is also a political matter.

Even at the time of the League of Nations, standards for the protection of human rights were laid down only in national constitutions. Hence, efforts were made within the United Nations to draft an international treaty which would make it possible to accuse a given state of a violation of human rights. After this had proved impossible, there was general agreement on a *Universal Declaration of Human Rights* which was adopted by the General Assembly of the United Nations on December 10, 1948. The rights proclaimed in the Declaration have been set forth in two Covenants adopted by the General Assembly on December 16, 1966. These were the 'International Covenant on Civil and Political Rights', supplemented by an Optional Protocol providing measures of implementation, and the 'International Covenant of Economic, Social and Cultural Rights', both entered into force in 1976. The Declaration, together with the two Covenants and the Optional Protocol constitute the *International Bill of Human Rights*.

No doubt that human rights likewise are rights of children and so far we find the identical principles within the Bill of Human Rights. But during childhood and adolescence the human being needs special protection. Therefore it is necessary to recognize and to define the special rights and obligations of minors.

THE RIGHTS OF THE CHILD

As early as 1924 the League of Nations adopted the 'Geneva Declaration of the Rights of the Child' which, however, evoked only a limited response. Efforts had been made since 1948 within the United Nations to achieve a broader and improved version of this document and, as a result, the General Assembly on November 20, 1959 adopted and proclaimed the *Declaration of the Rights of the Child*. On December 21, 1976, in anticipation of the twentieth anniversary of this declaration, the General Assembly resolved to provide a new incentive towards the improvement of the situation of children throughout the world by proclaiming 1979 to be the 'Year of the Child'.

At the same time the Commission on Human Rights began to work on the drafting of a convention, an international treaty, on the rights of the child. The substance of the present draft is based essentially on the Declaration of 1959. But in terms of legal consequences there are significant differences between an international treaty and a declaration. Therefore justified criticism was voiced, e.g., about the mixing of provisions dealing with the rights of the individual with those concerned with the obligations and duties of the State.

This raises the question whether it is meaningful and practical to create an international treaty agreement which reaches beyond the scope of a formal declaration. Bearing in mind the limited courses of action available to the United Nations in matters of human rights violations, one will tend to be sceptical. It must be borne in mind after all that the essential rights of the child, the violation of which could provide the basis of an action within the framework of the Commission for Human Rights, are already set forth in the provisions and agreements of the International Bill of Human Rights which has been referred to earlier.

Let us now look more closely at some of these provisions, firstly the *Universal Declaration of Human Rights*. According to Article 16, Paragraph 3, the family is the natural and fundamental group unit of society and is entitled to protection by society and the State. This statement is extended in Article 25, Paragraph 2: "Motherhood and childhood are entitled to special care and assistance. All children, whether born in or out of wedlock, shall enjoy the same social protection." In addition, Article 26, Paragraph 3 states: "Parents have a prior right to choose the kind of education that shall be given to their children."

Thus we already have a number of statements which could be the subject of very lengthy discussion. We are concerned here with the relationship between the family and State, the rights of parents as a constitutional norm, the possibilities of the State and their limits, i.e. the power to control and regulate the rights of parents to determine the education of their children, in other words the power of the State to govern through its organs the life of the family. Naturally, no one will dispute the fact that, in cases of obvious inability of parents to meet their educational obligations for whatever reasons, the State has the duty to take the necessary steps on behalf of the child.

However, when we are dealing with the *borderline zone* barely capable of specific definition opinions may well differ as to whether the intervention of the State would better serve the interests of the child. More recent legislation in various states is concerned with such questions and has offered various solutions. As far as the Federal Republic of Germany is concerned we might make reference to the recent *Parental Care Act* of July 18, 1979 (BGB1. I, 1061) and the draft bill on *Assistance to Juveniles* which is still the object of parliamentary discussion.

In Articles 10 and 13 of the *International Covenant on Economic, Social and Cultural Rights*, the provisions of the Declaration of Human Rights, to which we have made reference, are specified and supplemented. There is explicit emphasis on the importance and need for protection of the family as the "natural and fundamental group unit of society". It is recognized that Party States have to adopt appropriate measures for the *protection of the mother* as well as special measures, i.e. legal provisions, for the *protection of juveniles from economic and social exploitation.*

In the current discussion of educational reform in general and school reform in particular the provisions of Article 13, Paragraph 3, deserve special mention. These obligate the Party States to respect the liberty of parents and legal guardians "to choose for their children schools, others than those established by the public authorities" and "to ensure the religious and moral education of their children in conformity with their own conviction".

Here, too, is a topic for a very lengthy discussion. To what extent is the State permitted and to what extent must it regulate school and university education, in certain circumstances without regard to the more or less justified wishes of individual groups of parents or legal guardians?

Article 23 of the *International Covenant on Civil and Political Rights* again emphasizes the importance of marriage and the family and their right to special protection by the State and Society. The Party States shall, by appropriate measures, ensure the *equality of rights and responsibilities of spouses.* It also states: "In the case of dissolution, provision shall be made for the necessary protection of any children". According to Article 24 every child, without regard to race or colour, has the right to such measures of protection as are required by his status as a minor, on the part of his family, society and the State.

A series of provisions in this covenant is concerned with the administration of justice, with jurisdiction and the execution of prison sentences. Article 10, Paragraph 2b states that an accused juvenile person shall be separated from adults and brought as speedily as possible for adjudication. Paragraph 3 states: "Juvenile offenders shall be segregated from adults and be accorded treatment appropriate to their age and legal status". And finally Article 14, Paragraph 4 states: "In the case of juvenile persons, the procedure shall be such as will take account of their age and the desirability of promoting their rehabilitation".

These provisions also raise a number of questions which cannot be dealt with in detail here. These examples are designed merely to demonstrate that we already have an international treaty agreement, which provides the framework within which violations of general human rights as well as violations of specific rights of the child can be questioned through the procedures of the Commission on Human Rights. Resolution 1503 (XLVIII) of May 27, 1970, passed by the Social and Economic Council, made the procedure considerably more effective but it is still longwinded and problematical. The '1503-Procedure' has nevertheless made it possible in the case of "a consistent pattern of gross and reliably attested violations of human rights" to take certain measures and make recommendations, although these must always be within the framework of what is politically feasible at the international level. The provisions of this procedure have somewhat limited the principle of the sovereignty of states, referred to above, or at any rate where there is within a state a 'situation' which appears to reveal a consistent pattern of gross and reliably attested violations of human rights and fundamental freedoms.

This all sounds very complicated and difficult but, according to the Report of the General Secretary to the General Assembly, 47 777 communications were dealt with by this procedure during the period from June 1, 1975 to April 30, 1976. This figure is surprisingly high and provides food for thought. It is impossible to say anything specific about the results of these procedures, since all such action is regarded as confidential and thus details are not available to the public.

As well as individual communications about a violation of human rights, there are communications by a state to the effect that another state is not fulfilling its obligations under the Covenant as is set forth in Article 41 of the Covenant on Civil and Political Rights. The principle of reciprocity applies here, i.e. communications may be received and considered only if they are submitted by a state which has made a declaration recognizing the competence of the Committee, as provided for in Article 41, and with regard to a state which has made a similar declaration. For the moment it is impossible to say how this provision will work in practice. The covenant is new and at present only a few states have made the required declaration.

CURRENT PRACTICAL QUESTIONS

The system of international declarations, agreements and treaties on the subject of human rights in general and the rights of the child in particular, created within the framework of the activities of the United Nations, is extensive and complicated. Mention should also be made here of the *Declaration on Rights of Mentally Retarded Persons* of 1971 and the *Declaration on Rights of Disabled Persons* in general of 1975. Hence one căn only note with slight astonishment that, in this 'Year of the Child', work proceeds with surprising intensity, at various levels, on general and fundamental declarations of the rights of the child, whilst no reference is made to what has already been achieved in this field within the United Nations. There seems to me to be an urgent necessity for us to concentrate our attention and activities more on the concrete problems which arise in practice.

Under the aspects of mental health, consideration should be given to such matters as:

- rights of the unborn and abortion;
- coming of age and criminal responsibility;
- abuse of alcohol and drugs;
- ill-treatment of children and child labour;
- relation between rights and obligations of children and of parents with respect to the family as the basic unit of society.

Each of these topics could be the subject of a large paper or book, and the complicated problems involved cannot be dealt with in detail here. In many countries we have legal regulations for the protection of children and of families. Some are good, many insufficient. But in matters of human rights in general and of rights of children in detail we should not expect too much from official declarations, from laws and administrative activities. Primarily we are confronted here with questions of education, especially of parents and of educators in the proper understanding of mental health in childhood and adolescence. Growing up in the changing world of today means: opening the doors for the minor to recognize and to accept a system of values and standards, not only to pose questions.

Director,
University Institute of Forensic and Social Psychiatry,
Marburg, W. Germany

REFERENCES

Allen, R. C.
1969 Legal Rights of the Disabled and Disadvantaged. Washington.
Baldwin, A. L.
1967 Theories of child development. New York.
Beizke, G.
1978 Familienrecht. 19. Aufl., Muenchen.
Ehrhardt, H. E.
1972 Drug Abuse in Europe: Medical and Legal Aspects. In: Drug Abuse (ed. W. Keup), Springfield, p. 27.
1975 Abortion and Euthanasia. The Human Life Review (New York), Vol. 1, Nr. 3, p. 12.
1976 Die artifizielle Insemination. IV. World Congress on Medical Law, Manila. Proceedings A.XII. Mschr. Krim 59, 173.
1978 Ethical Problems in Psychiatric Practice. VI. World Congress of Psychiatry. Psychiatric Annals (New York), 8, 21.
1979 Der zivilrechtliche Schutz psychisch Kranker and Behinderter, Arch. f. Wissensch.u. Praxis d.soz. Arbeit, 10, 171.
Ermacora, F.
1974 Menschenrechte im Wandel der Zeit Bd. I, Vienna.
Feltes, T.
1978 Jugendrecht im Konflikt zwischen Normen und Erziehung, Munich.
Hinz, M.
1976 Kinderschutz als Rechtsschutz, Paderborn.
Luard, E. (ed.)
1967 The International Protection of Human Rights, London.
Meissner, F.
1976 Die Menschenrechtsbeschwerde vor den Vereinten Nationen, Baden-Baden.
Morrison, C. C.
1967 The developing European law of human rights. Leiden.
Noll-Wagenfeld, M.
1977 Aktionsmoeglichkeiten der Vereinten Nationen bei Menschenrechtsverletzungen, VN 6, p. 180.
Piaget, J.
1967 La psychologie de l'enfant, 26 ed., Paris.
Reuter, D.
1968 Kindesgrundrechte und elterliche Gewalt, Berlin.
Schreiber, M.
1975 La pratique recente des Nations Unies dans le domaine de la protection des droits de l'homme. Recueil des Cours de la Haye II, p. 315.

Schwelb, E.
1972 Zur Frage der Anrufung der UN-Menschenrechtskommission durch Individuen und nichtstaatliche Organisationen, VN 3, S. 79.
Sohn, L. B. and Buergenthal, T.
1973 International Protection of Human Rights, Indianapolis.
Steigerwald, R. (Hrsg.)
1977 Menschenrechte in der Diskussion, Vienna.
Tomuschat, C.
1976 Menschenrechtschutz durch die Vereinten Nationen, VN 6, S. 166.
Verdooth, A.
1964 Naissance et signification de la declaration universelle des droits de l'homme, Paris.

Mrs. HILDA H. ROBBINS, B.S. (Ec.) (U.S.A.)

SECURING RIGHTS OF CHILDREN BY CITIZEN ADVOCACY

The Mental Health Association in the United States has been active for many years in securing those Rights of Children which are particularly associated with mental health and mental illness. The experiences and observations of this paper are those of one who has been an active, vocal, participating volunteer in the Mental Health Association for twenty-five years. They are shared in the spirit and hope that all children may come closer to full enjoyment of all their rights.

An enumeration of some of the crimes against and indignities suffered by children and a review of the Rights of Children as listed by four different sources provides a basis for examination of the advocacy activities of the Mental Health Association in the United States.

A few of the hurts heaped upon our children every day include:

(1) Children suffer physical abuse – sometimes leading to death. Thousands of children are killed by their own parents – and 200 000 are seriously abused in the U.S. each year.

(2) Children suffer emotional deprivation and mental illness. In the United states we know that 15% of our children need mental health services – but only 10% receive adequate mental health services.

(3) Children suffer physical illness and physical handicaps. But less than 10% of the government health money in the United States is spent on children.

(4) Children suffer because the mentally and physically handicapped receive inferior educational and recreational opportunities.

(5) Children suffer starvation and malnutrition. This contributes to early and lifelong physical and mental problems.

(6) Children suffer incarceration in adult jails, prisons, *and* hospitals. Many such involuntary confinements are made without legal counsel or due process.

(7) Children suffer from inadequate information about sex and reproduction. Children bearing children is economically untenable and emotionally baffling. An unloved child often becomes an unloving adult.

(8) Children suffer from punitive confinement, overmedication and aversive behavior therapy.

(9) Children suffer when parents work and no safe and professionally staffed day care center is available.

(10) Children suffer when parents separate or divorce and custody laws

S. H. Fine, R. Krell, and Tsung-yi Lin (Eds.), 'Today's Priorities in Mental Health', 85–92.

are unfair and unenforceable. Using children as pawns is a travesty of parental responsibility.

I believe all these hurtful conditions are worldwide.

Some people like to believe there was a time when child neglect and abuse did not exist – when parents could be trusted to be the sole benevolent protectors of their children. Not so! History is filled with periods of organized and condoned child abuse and exploitation. In most nations parenthood remains the greatest single preserve of the amateur. Listing 'The Rights of Children' in formal documents is the first step in correction.

One of the early and significant documents of the United Nations was a Declaration of the Rights of Children. In 1948 they issued a list of children's rights which have been repeated with minor modifications in all subsequent lists of children's rights. That list of ten included the right:

to adequate nutrition and medical care
to affection, love and understanding
to be a useful member of society
to a name and a nationality
to be brought up in a spirit of peace and universal brotherhood
to free education
to full opportunity for play and recreation
to special care if handicapped
to be among the first to receive relief in time of disaster
to enjoy these rights regardless of race, color, sex, religion, national or social origin

The 'Right to special care if handicapped' has always had a very significant meaning to the National Mental Health Association, and one of the continuing efforts has been to gain recognition and care for those children without visible handicaps. Most children with emotional problems do not receive early recognition nor do they receive early and periodic screening, diagnosis and treatment. Our Association has been working in coalition with 25 other organizations to secure these services. Over 500 of our volunteers have made contacts with national lawmakers on this issue. These efforts have caused significant improvements in the Childhood Health Assessment Program. But our efforts will continue because services for the emotionally ill child still are less than for the physically ill child.

The White House Conference of 1930 was a landmark event for mentally ill children. There, for the first time, the emotionally disturbed child was identified as having special needs and deserving special treatment and claiming special rights. At another White House Conference on Children in 1970 a list of rights central to a child's well-being was categorized into six basic rights. Of those six rights, the Mental Health Association has been particularly involved in "the right to be educated to the limits of one's capabilities." We worked for several years to finally get the passage of a law in 1975 called the 'Education of All Handicapped Children Law.' The law is technical and complicated and our Association continues to act as an advocate to help interpret the law, to stimulate schools to comply with it, and to get adequate funding.

The *Joint Commission on the Mental Health of Children* made a 3 year study. The report from the Commission, *Crisis in Child Mental Health; Challenge for the 70s*, was widely read and the 7 basic rights which were identified have been printed often, quoted often, and ignored often.

From this list the Mental Health Association has focused on getting adequate and appropriate care and treatment as a top priority. The Association has a strong and vocal Children's Committee including advocates whose children are consumers of mental health services, and many who are relatives, friends, judges, teachers and others who live with and love troubled children.

With the funding of Community Mental Health Centers in 1964 there was great hope that emotionally disturbed children would at least be served. However, site evaluations and visits by members of the Mental Health Association across the country found that many centers provided no services for children. This situation was brought to the attention of lawmakers and sufficient pressure was applied by our members to get changes requiring more children's services. By 1975 about 23% of all the people being seen in centers were under 18 years of age. However, there are still millions of children and adolescents, disturbed and hurting, and not receiving care. In some areas services still do not exist; in some areas there are services but there is discrimination; in some areas the service is poor and youngsters are misdiagnosed and mislabeled, removed from their homes and communities and confined to hospital wards with psychotic adults or to other depersonalized institutions which deliver little more than custodial care. Irving N. Berlin writing in *Advocacy for Child Mental Health* in 1975 expanded on the Commission's 7 basic rights by adding the right to meaningful employment, ethnic identity, and political participation. He placed great emphasis on the fact that poverty and racism continue to be major societal, health, and mental health problems.

The National Mental Health Association has also prepared a list of children's rights. They are illustrated and explained in English and Spanish in a pamphlet called *What Every Child Needs*. The volunteers and staff of the Mental Health Association identified the right to:

Love
Security
Acceptance
Control/Limits
Guidance
Independence

Protection
Faith

This pamphlet has been widely distributed through our public information service. The lists referred to are appended to this paper in a chart form for easy reference.

Why is it necessary to specifically identify children's rights? Children are almost totally voiceless and powerless in claiming their rights, defending their rights and their persons, and in getting access to redress for damages to themselves. Surely this is worldwide.

Many children at some time need the intervention and assistance of adults with power. They need help from adults other than family or those who provide various services. Who are those adults with power who can help children who are hurting? In the United States the most consistently successful efforts on behalf of children have been initiated by well organized special interest groups who are avid advocates. These are not advocates in the traditional legal meaning of the word. Most of these advocates are volunteers who are not professionals. They are consumer-citizens with a common concern who know the constructive use of power.

Regrettably this type of advocacy is *not* worldwide nor is it as widely practiced in the United States as it needs to be.

The United States has a history of involvement between government and voluntary organizations, and there is a constant vigilance to maintain a balance that does not diminish the freedom and flexibility of the voluntary sector. The Mental Health Association is a good example of an effective voluntary organization which has learned some successful techniques for bringing about social change in our social system. What is workable and useful in this system may need to be modified to be applicable in other systems. The Mental Health Association has fought to expand and liberalize the right to be a true consumer advocacy agency.

Four years ago a massive and prolonged effort by over 350 grass roots organizations led by the Mental Health Association resulted in removing major legal and statutory restraints then limiting our lobbying activities. This had freed the Association to give substantially more time to influencing legislation. It took 5 years to get this legislative change.

The Mental Health Association has upwards of a million volunteer members in 850 affiliated associations. About 90% of these volunteers are not mental health professionals. Since we were founded in 1909 by Clifford Beers who was a consumer of mental health services, we have always identified ourselves and used our voice as 'advocate for mentally ill persons and their families.' This role means that our activities may cover a wide variety of concerns and interests.

In addition to the Children and Adolescents Committee, we have other program committees including Ethnic Minorities, Research, Legislation and

Services. During the year members of each of these committees will be drafting legislation, monitoring legislation that is in the process of implementation, collecting data for budget recommendations, testifying before Congress, and preparing the briefing papers on one or more bills so that all our MHA members can make informed and persuasive contacts with their own lawmakers.

The Litigation Panel of the Association is one of our most potent tools for advocacy. This group of lawyers and lay persons reviews an average of 50 cases each year. In the last 8 years we have taken part in 19 cases. We recently lost an important case when the Supreme Court of the United States, in June 1979, decided that a child is not required to be given a full due-process-of-law hearing prior to being committed to a mental institution by the child's parents. This is a description of the components and some of the activities of only the advocacy arm of our Association. Of course all our members, including those involved in other departments such as communications, organization, and development, are also enthusiastic lobbyists when called to action.

There are a few characteristics of the Mental Health Association which have helped it grow in strength and influence as an advocacy agency. They have been important to us and may be helpful to others.

We insist that we are *the* citizen-advocate organization in mental health. This has fostered a rather tenacious independence.

We hold to our independence when pressured to merge with other organizations.

We strongly defend our independence as a social action agency and not a service provider organization.

We steadfastly retain our independence from professional organizations and providers of service. Leadership roles are always held by non-professionals.

We volunteers guard rather zealously our independence from domination by our own dedicated professional staff. Policy is set by the volunteers and then the team of staff and volunteers join in carrying it forward.

But by far our hardest and most important struggle is to maintain independence from the government. With inflation, it becomes increasingly difficult to resist the seduction of public dollars. But the National Mental Health Association has adopted a quite restrictive policy regarding acceptance of government funds. It is felt that our credibility is compromised and financial stability is jeopardized by accepting government dollars. Less than 1% of our budget has been from government funds during the last ten years – and that for special projects. It requires a special effort to maintain this independence; however, it multiplies our power and establishes our integrity many times over.

In addition to these characteristics of our Association we have found a few principles most important in building a strong volunteer advocacy association.

First, effective citizen action requires stamina. To have impact requires sustained effort. As an example, at one time we had to get Congressional support to override two presidential vetoes to keep the Community Mental Health Centers alive. This meant twenty months of high-level pressure to be successful.

Second, effective citizen action requires focus. We must constantly say 'no' to requests which would divert us from our planned agenda. We know we must specifically and narrowly decide which policy decisions must be effected by the Mental Health Association, then focus our action. We take on only those issues we intend to fight through to conclusion. This year the Children's Committee has focused almost exclusively on the Childhood Health Assessment Program.

Third, effective citizen action requires that we understand how the government and the maze of health and mental health systems within it are organized and how they are changed. High-mindedness and blind emotion are no substitute for citizen skill. Programs affecting the lives of children are fragmented in over 100 different departments.

Fourth, effective citizen action requires accurate and carefully analyzed quantifiable data. Credibility with officials and credibility with the press are essential and must be protected.

Fifth, effective citizen action requires a sense of strategy development. Knowing how to build a coalition, identify the opposition, and measure the strengths and weaknesses of all parties is necessary social practical politics.

Sixth, effective citizen action requires close collaboration between the Mental Health Association professional staff and volunteers who have lead responsibility. The relationship between our professional staff and our volunteers is much like co-workers in similar professional positions. The trust and teamwork make for effective advocacy.

Using these principles, our citizen advocate association has found a way to make constructive use of adult consumer power – a power with the ability to cause change.

Much has been written about the use and abuse of power. What is the real meaning of power? Very simply, power is the ability to cause or prevent change. President Theodore Roosevelt said, "Our chief usefulness to humanity rests on our combining power with high purpose. Power undirected by high purpose spells calamity, and high purpose by itself is utterly useless if the power to put it into effect is lacking."

During 1979 thousands of Mental Health Association citizen volunteers and staff have been working on the most significant piece of mental health legislation since the creation of the community mental health program in 1963. This legislation is based on recommendations of the President's Commission on Mental Health made in 1978. Rosalynn Carter, the President's wife, was honorary chairperson of this Commission and was totally involved in all its hearings and in its recommendations. She was the first person to testify before Senator Kennedy's Committee regarding the legislation. There she firmly and convincingly stated, "I am an advocate for the mentally ill." Her intelligence, her compassion, and her prestige make her a powerful advocate indeed for all mentally ill. We are proud that she has been a contributing board member of our Association for 5 years. This new legislation is targeted to ensure mental health services for priority population groups including children, the elderly, the long-term mentally ill, minorities, and the poor and the other unserved groups.

Cicero said, "Freedom is participation in power." The members of our Association have been practicing and learning and enjoying some measure of that freedom as our activities as an advocate organization have grown steadily since 1950. Nearly all the progress made so far in establishing the legal rights of children and the mentally ill has come in the last decade. But we know that laws and legal rights do not enforce themselves. The mentally ill need their own independent and skilled advocates if they are not to be exploited. The Association is now helping to write legislation for an external advocacy system designated specifically and only for the mentally ill. It would provide a permanent, independent, qualified, official and professional resource and support system for eliminating the discrimination against the mentally ill – including children. This would in no way take the place of volunteer advocates. It is our voices which will make the difference – not the cries of hurting children.

John Gardner is one of our most eloquent and effective citizens on behalf of consumer advocacy. A dramatic poster was designed with his words which inspired many. It said: "Nations decay, only the citizens, critical and loving, can bring them back to life."

Margaret Mead also had a clear concept of both the necessity and the power of volunteer activism. She said, "Only by involving adults, all adults – adults who have never had children and adults whose children have grown up – can we hope to combine reform in the care of specific groups of children – deaf children, crippled children, orphaned children – with a genuine attempt to rethink the way our towns and cities are built and the way our lives are lived."

President,
National Mental Health Association, U. S. A.
Arlington,
Virginia,
U. S. A.

Rights for Children

Joint Commission on the Mental Health of Children	U.N. Declaration of the Rights of the Child	What every child needs – Mental Health Association	1970 White House Conference on Children
The right to be born wanted.	The right to affection, love and understanding.	Love	The right to grow in a society which respects the dignity of life and is free of poverty, discrimination, and other forms of degradation.
The right to be born healthy.	The right to adequate nutrition and medical care.	Security	The right to be born and be healthy and wanted through childhood.
The right to live in a healthful environment.	The right to free education.	Acceptance	The right to grow up nurtured by affectionate parents.
The right to (satisfaction of) basic needs.	The right to full opportunity for play and recreation.	Control (Limits)	The right to be a child during childhood, to have meaningful choices in the process of maturation and development, and to have a meaningful voice in the community.
The right to continuous and loving care.	The right to a name and nationality.	Guidance	The right to be educated to the limits of one's capability and through processes designed to elicit one's full potential.
The right to acquire intellectual and emotional skills (To achieve individual aspirations to cope effectively in our society).	The right to special care, if handicapped.	Independence	The right to have societal mechanisms to enforce the foregoing rights.
The right to (receive care and) treatment through facilities which are appropriate to (their) needs and which keep them as closely as possible within their normal social setting.	The right to be among the first to receive relief in times of disaster.	Protection	
	The right to be a useful member of society and to develop individual abilities.	Faith	
	The right to be brought up in a spirit of peace and universal brotherhood.		
	The right to enjoy these rights, regardless of race, color, sex, religion, national or social origin.		

QUENTIN RAE-GRANT, M.B., Ch.B., F.R.C.Psych., F.R.C.P. (C) (Canada)

CHILDREN'S RIGHTS

The rights accorded to children either in law or in moral and ethical practices are a reflection of the status of the child in a particular society at a particular time. They are continually evolving, although not always in a smooth and desirable progression. It most cases they cannot be legislated, as legislation can only effectively canonize that which society has already accepted. The advocacy for children's rights is generally spearheaded by groups who are out of step with the majority of society and who propose changes that are initially briskly resisted, then reluctantly accepted, and in retrospect are seen as manifestly justified. The task then is twofold: To advance in new areas while securing society's acceptance and, simultaneously to protect the gains that have already been made. The rhetoric can exhort to the utopian; the practical goal is to achieve what society will realistically implement, while laying the groundwork for further protections.

This presentation would like, therefore, to look at the question of children's rights from a historical and developmental perspective, admittedly relying mostly on European and North American developments, to underline how far we have come and to avoid self-recriminatory expostulations. It would be hoped that this would illustrate how far we have come, the distance we still have to go, and the problems that can be created in effectively implementing changes in practice that parallel the laudable benefits of the theory. The task is major; the time is ripe for further advances and changes. No time is more auspicious than this Year of the Child; no task is more appropriate for support from a group such as the World Federation for Mental Health.

In his Presidential Address in 1961 to the American Orthopsychiatric Association, Dr. Fritz Redl described the child's real position in North American society which had prided itself on its concerned care of young people. His statement that society operated on the basis of "the love of kids, neglect of children, hatred of youth" was a graphic attempt to arouse the conscience of the mental health establishment to the gap between aspiration and practice (Redl 1962) (Hospital and Community Psychiatry 1975). The Joint Commission on the Mental Health of Children elaborated on the same theme:

> We proclaim that we are a nation devoted to its young. We believe that we have made great strides toward recognizing the needs of children and youth. We have enacted labour laws, established a public education system, created treatment services for our disturbed and handicapped, and devised imaginative programs such as Head Start for our disadvantaged young. Yet we find ourselves dismayed by the violence, frustration and discontent among our youth and by the sheer number of emotionally, mentally, physically and socially handi-

S. H. Fine, R. Krell, and Tsung-yi Lin (Eds.), 'Today's Priorities in Mental Health' 93–105.

capped youngsters in our midst. It is shocking to know that thousands of children are still excluded from our schools, that millions in need go untreated, and that many still suffer from hunger and malnutrition. (Joint Commission on Mental Health of Children 1970).

There is little need to expand. We can all recognize the great attention paid to the adolescent and youth population with its enormous purchasing potential – an attention which empahsizes material goods, possessions, and conspicuous consumption. In the late '60s, in the era of advocacy, there was a substantial liberalization of both practice and adage particularly towards emancipated youth, but when the pressure declined these precarious gains were subject to attrition. Though several jurisdictions, indeed countries, agreed that the use of marijuana was dangerous (mostly insofar as it involved infractions of the legal code and potential severe penalties therefrom) it is disappointing to know how few, if any, have taken the logical step of making its use and possession a non-illegal activity. This has the further complication of producing a contempt and challenge for laws when well over half the population in these age groups are known to use it.

Indeed the formal legal rights of the child are still very few. They are basically the right to adequate nutrition, housing, protection from physical abuse and gross neglect, the right to education and an emerging right to be heard in decisions which affect his or her own future. All other rights reside in the parent or the guardian and are subject to the goodwill or the idiosyncratic whim of these individuals. Those of us who care for or treat children have not been as vigilant as we might. We have stoutly maintained that there should be no differentiation between physical and emotional illness and yet we stand by or have to accept the relative unavailability of services for such life-threatening situations as attempted suicide, acute psychotic episodes, or potential child abuse. In most areas, even in the best developed, our system of caring and treatment remains a patchy, unintegrated, frequently competitive array of disconnected services (Central Toronto Youth Services 1975) (Hobbs 1975) (Kittrie 1971) (Rafferty 1964). Even of more concern is that at times we justify what is being done to the child without consulting him, as in our opinion it is in the child's best interests. We can admit, retain, impose sanctions on him in the name of treatment and rehabilitation which, because they become practice, have simply bypassed the processes of continual consideration and scrutiny. Adults in the U.S. have both the right to treatment and the right to refuse treatment. Children and adolescents have neither. But lest we slip once again into the trap of losing our perspective, let us briefly review the historical status and see how far we have come, without being smug about progress.

Four main divisions in the state of the child can be discussed from the times of the Greeks and Romans to modern day society:

1. Child as non-existent – where the status of the child was as a part of patriarchial worldly wealth.
2. Child as co-existent – the child as munchkin, undistinguished from the adult except by size.

3. Child as pet – where the child was a voiceless faithful companion to be trained, or an object to be profited by or neglected.
4. Child as person, but only tentatively – the phase we have entered where the child's rights are being respected by some of the people some of the time, but only under certain specific adult-defined conditions.

(1) Perhaps the mood of early times is best captured in a quote from Aristotle: "The justice of a master or a father is a different thing from that of a citizen, for a son or slave is property and there can be no injustice to one's own property" (*Harvard Ed. Rev.* 1973). In the father resided total power over the child under the logical resolutions that "he who gave life also had the power of taking it away" (Russell unpublished). *Patriae Potestas*, the life and death policy, was practiced by Persians, Egyptians, Greeks and Gauls.

In Sparta and Athens, children whom the father considered not worth hanging onto were exposed to the elements and wild animals to die (Despert 1965). These children included the illegitimate, those too sickly to be worth anything to the father, and surplus children conceived after the father had decided that his family was large enough. With the coming of Christianity to the Roman Empire, the power of the father was somewhat mitigated and the decision of life and death came to rest with the State.

Norman-conquest England recognized the dictum of *Parens Patriae* which allowed that "the State has ultimate rights of guardianship over persons under legal disability to protect themselves – the idiots, deranged, insane, lepers and children." (Russell unpublished).

In 1275 the German law (The Munt) recognized the right of the father to sell a child in case of necessity (Russell unpublished). As late as 1646 a Massachusetts Bay Colony statute proclaimed that if a father had a son who was "rebellious or stubborn of at least 16 years of age", the child could be brought to magistrate's court where "such a son shall be put to death" (Time Magazine 1972).

(2) Even when the child was recognized as an immature co-existent, childhood was seen to extend only until he could cope and verbalize. Mystically, at age 7 the child became an adult. The child was ignored until that age and then trained as quickly as possible to be an adult.

Childhood, then, was not considered a stage of development but an age of incapacity, unlinked by any kind of continuity with adulthood. In the paintings of the middle ages, children were depicted as smaller versions of adults, anatomically undistinguished except by size (Aries 1970). Until the 17th century they were not even accorded the privilege of different dress (Aries 1970). They moved from swaddling clothes to suits of armour. Although the first recognition was the abominable knickers, at least it did mark the first tentative step towards today's mandatory denim uniform. Even from a medical point of view, the child remained unrecognized until the 16th century when the first pediatric books were written (Despert 1965).

(3) Perhaps the third stage is best encapsulated by the petulant complaints about the attention that children were increasingly receiving. Montagne bristles, "I cannot abide that passion for caressing newborn children which have neither mental activities nor recognizable bodily shape by which to make themselves lovable, and have never wittingly suffered them to be fed in my presence" (Aries 1970). The ideas of people like Montagne ran counter to the ambivalence of the Middle Ages: "They held that it was no longer desirable that children should mingle with adults, especially at the table. No doubt because if they did, they were spoiled and became ill-mannered".

Then an even greater upheaval changed child upbringing – the movement to universal education.

"Henceforth it was recognized", says Aries, "that the child was not ready for life and that he had to be subjected to a special treatment, a sort of quarantine, before he was allowed to join the adults" (Aries 1970).

Finally, at least in some ways, the society of adults had begun to admit the existence of the society of children. In the late 19th and early 20th centuries, the issue of child rights began finding its way into the courts. Sweeping advances for the causes of children were made: new labor laws, educational laws, the inception of juvenile courts; orphanages were set up to house the child of the streets. Yet, looking back, much of what was done was misdirected, more abusive at times than useful, and often 'too little too late' (Bremner 1971). The adult began to grant a new and heretofore unrecognized role to the child, that of a separate but, as yet, incompetent being. For the child of rich parents this meant that a nanny governed his/her life until age 7 or so when a private boarding school would see them through until they became acceptable to be received 'upon their debut' into the adult world. For these favoured children, no civil rights movement was prompted much less anticipated by the adult populace. The benefactor of the humanitarian rush to do 'in his best interests' was the child of the barn, beating, and bootblack.

Perhaps the first indication of the child's new status was the creation of societies to protect and preserve the child from immoral or abusive elements. The first society to be organized in the U.S. was the Society for the Prevention of Cruelty to Children – an outgrowth of the Society for the Prevention of Cruelty to Animals (Bremner 1971). Despite its name, the New York S.P.C.C. was not as much interested or involved in the prevention of cruelty as in the rescue of children from improper homes, the enforcement of laws, and the punishment of offenders against children (Bremner 1971). Twenty-five years after this Society's beginning in 1874, there were 250 societies in the U.S. (Bremner 1971). In the eyes of these early Children's Aid Societies, there was one solution for a poor, orphaned, neglected or abused 'waif' – placement in the benevolent institution. This push ensured that the institutionalized child was hermetically sealed from the world, protected from misdirecting and miscorrecting indigent adults (Rae-Grant and Moffat 1971) (Celdic 1970).

At the same time home-finding societies sprang up. These two types of caring organizations could not work together – one taking the child off the streets; one placing him in a secure family environment. "Indifference on the part of the officials, pride in numbers, and a funding system that only paid money to institutions ensured the prolongation of institutional care" (Bremner 1971).

With societal separation came criminal separation and in 1892 a criminal code amendment was passed in Canada which asserted that children should have a different trial from adults, one that stressed correction and privacy (Solicitor General's Committee 1975). Unlike adult court, the juvenile process espoused a more liberal choice of disposition, and emphasis was shifted towards a therapeutic mode. The intent was to provide a more humane processing, one that was to be 'in the best interests of the child'. In return for this privilege, ironically, the child was stripped of most of the liberties of the adult court. He was not accorded the right to bail, to counsel, or the right to confront his accusers (Kittrie 1971). A review opinion 60 years later reads:

> The original Juvenile Court Act as enacted . . . was devised to afford the juvenile protections *in addition* to those he already possessed. . . . Before this legislative enactment, the juvenile was subject to the same punishment for an offence as an adult. It follows logically that in the absence of such legislation the juvenile would be entitled to the same constitutional guarantees and safeguards as an adult. If this be true then the only possible reason for the Juvenile Court Act was to afford the juvenile safeguards in addition to those he already possessed. The legislature's intent was to enlarge, not to diminish, these protections. (1955) (Kittrie 1971). [The effect was the opposite.]

At about the same time as Juvenile Acts were being passed, a crusade against child labor began. The new psychology had proclaimed that playtime was an important part of creating whole adults. R. Hunter puts it, "You cannot rob children of their play any more than you can forget and neglect the children at their play as we now do in the tenement district without at the same time paying the penalty. When children are robbed of playtime, they too often reassert their right to it in manhood as vagabonds, criminals and prostitutes" (Bremner 1971).

One fact unites all of the changes procured for the child in the early 19th and 20th centuries. Each change was undertaken with good intentions and always justified as done in the best interests of the child. Thus in the early 1900s, a case appeared before the courts in which a child, Lulu Roller, brought a charge of rape against her father to the Supreme Court of Washington State. The case was thrown out of court. The grounds for dismissal? In the judge's words, "The rule of law prohibiting suits between parent and child is based on the interest that society has in preserving harmony in the domestic relations" (Time Magazine 1972). The child still was not recognized as an entity in himself, a being who to varying degrees is capable of expressing his own wishes and preferences. The child is tied to his parents by an umbilical cord that stretches into custody proceedings, juvenile court hearings, and medical treatment.

As William Arkman said in 1972, "The child's legal status is an amalgamation of non-citizen, slave, over-protected pet and valuable chattel" (Canadian Mental Health Association (Quebec) 1974).

In the last few years, a subtle change has begun to take place again in the status of the child. The change is slow to come, and many who are not concerned directly with the area are still unaware of its inception. The change is an admission on the adult world's part that the child has one further basic right, a right that filters into every area of childhood concern – the home, school and court – the right to be heard (Canadian Mental Health Association (Quebec) 1974) (Marker and Friedman 1973).

The landmark case of the new move for children was the Gault case (Wittenberg 1976). Gerald Gault was sentenced to 7 years in industrial school for prank calls in which he made "remarks or questions of the irritatingly offensive adolescent sex variety". The alarming and contagious content consisted of the following questions: "Do you give any? Are your cherries ripe today? Do you have big bombers?" If he were 16, he would have gone to jail for only two months. As it was, it took a Writ of Habeas Corpus, two years, and a trip to the Supreme Court before he was released in 1967 (Kittrie 1971). The ruling in this case extended to juveniles many of the legal rights that adults are granted – the right to counsel, the right to cross-examine and confront hostile witnesses, the right to avoid self-incrimination (Bremner 1971). This was perhaps the first instance where juveniles were declared to have the same right to be heard as adults.

Later decisions affected other areas of children's rights: "Although the authority of a parent is generally controlling, this does not mean . . . . that such authority is unlimited" (Melville *v*. Sabbatino, 313A. 2d886,888 (Conn. Super Ct. 1973)). "School officials do not have absolute authority over their students. State operated schools may not be enclaves of totalitarianism". (Tinker *v*. Des Moines Independent School District (393 U.S. 503)). "The U.S. Supreme Court rules that states cannot apply 'preponderance of evidence' standards in juvenile proceedings. Proof beyond reasonable doubt is required". (*In re* Winship, (397 U.S. 358)). "The child has the right over whether to continue education and how" (Wisconsin *v*. Voder (1972)).

These legal decisions are only the beginning and can be subverted by human ingenuity. A court decision that school children in the U.S. could wear armbands to protest the war in Vietnam implied the spirit of sanctioning conscientious dissent to children as part of the right of freedom of speech (Bremner 1971) (Kittrie 1971). But as poverty lawyer Ernest Aubry said, "If somebody goes to class with a button that says 'Chicano Power', the authorities immediately say 'Well, that's not a black armband' " (Time Magazine 1972). Similarly, as soon as the Gault decision had passed into state legislation, juvenile courts in many areas began to ask parents to sign waivers of rights, giving up right to counsel, to avoid self-incrimination, and all other rights that were so hard fought for (Kittrie 1971). Case law is not a solution for any number of injustices created in the world.

The child's legal rights, then, are the right not to be neglected, abused or ill-treated and the emerging right to be heard. All other rights derive from the parents or caretakers.

In this obvious vaccum a number of attempts have been made to enunciate a series of moral rights. The State of New York Youth Commission has produced a Children's Bill of Rights (State of New York Youth Commission) modelled on that of the United Nations, as have many other jurisdictions.

The Joint Commission on the Mental Health of Children has similarly compiled its list of rights:

> The right to be wanted, the right to be born healthy, the right to live in a healthy environment, the right to satisfaction of basic needs, the right to continuous loving care, the right to acquire the intellectual and emotional skills necessary to achieve individual aspirations and to cope effectively in our society, the right to receive care and treatment through facilities which are appropriate to their needs and which keep them as closely as possible within their normal social setting (Joint Commission on Mental Health of Children 1970).

But the problem is how to translate these laudable rights into operational practices (Fox 1974). To some extent this is being accomplished by quietly changing procedures. It is recognized in practice, though not in law, that treatment of the acute emergency can be done in the absence of available parental consent. It is recognized in practice but unprotected by law that contraceptive advice counseling, and psychological and psychiatric intervention can be negotiated by and provided to the emancipated adolescent, but the interpretation of this policy is strictly the prerogative of the practitioner (Fraser 1975).

Two main definitive avenues are available:

(A) External policying, namely, the passage of laws and regulations with concomitant mechanisms of licensing, inspection and, if necessary, court involvement.

(B) Internal policy operations where the organization itself recognizes the need for change and stays ahead of the imposition of external sanctions and intrusions (Guttman 1974).

Both approaches are prone to problems. The first can invoke elaborate, cumbersome, mostly inappropriate proceedings, reporting, guarantees and mountains of paperwork. It becomes an opportunity and an invitation for the exercise of ingenuity on the part of staff and institution to quietly tell the external authorities how to shove it. It can invoke a mounting proportion of time in dealing with paperwork and legislation requirements – time which could much better be spent on direct care of children (Sowell 1976). The second approach of internal policy modification also has its difficulties. The necessity for change may be unrecognized. It may run counter to the interests, customs and styles of the staff. It may conflict with those tablets of wisdom, the standing orders of the institution. However, it is clear that if policies do not change from within, change, often inappropriate, arbitrary, complex and confusing will undoubtedly be imposed from outside.

Let me try at this point to summarize and highlight some of the issues in the development of personal rights for children. Each time that a right is enunciated, other personal rights may inadvertently be sabotaged. This I have tried to illustrate in the juvenile delinquency area where the gain in the more humane approach was at the sacrifice of attention to the adjudication process and, because it was in the best interests of the child, not subject to appeal. In effect, then, for an offence which for an adult would have been minor, considerable disruption and intervention in the child's life was implemented and was felt to be justified. Of more concern is the repeated observation that the creation of a right may create a whole new set of problems.

Thus the right to universal education was almost always accompanied by compulsory attendance legislation. Truancy now became an offence; school avoidance or school phobia – the psychiatric diagnosis. Indeed, Werry *et al.* (Werry *et al.* 1972) have suggested that this may be one of the main causes of the present epidemic of learning disabilities. In the clinical practice area we can take legitimate pride in the development in recent years of a network of treatment services. However, in placing children in these treatment services we have been most cavalier with regard to their rights. As the study of Residential Care/Children in Canada says, "While residential programs are necessary, they are regrettable; it is regrettable that they are necessary" (Rae-Grant and Moffat 1971). Residential care is used when other resource people are disillusioned, angry, impotent or frankly scared and are grateful for any relief. At this point the last concern is the rights of the child; the primary concern is the passage of responsibility to some other agency. The already tenuous rights of children become even more rarified on admission, during residential stay, and on exit. If one defines a group of children in need of medical care, there are very few circumstances under which care is not available. Yet with psychiatric care there are roadblocks such as rather restrictive admission criteria, a careful selection of patients, avoidance of children who have simultaneous physical as well as emotional disorders, and a Monday-to-Friday office-hours schedule (Rae-Grant and Moffat 1971). I doubt whether anywhere there are enough facilities to respond to an adolescent emergency such as an attempted suicide which requires hospitalization. It is only recently that public concern has become aroused with regard to this situation.

The second area that again takes the child's rights and manipulates them is caused by different funding patterns in which the choice of the treatment program may be determined more by the financial auspices than by the child's needs (Celdic 1970) (Central Toronto Youth Services 1975) (Rae-Grant and Moffat 1971). The method of contracting with children for treatment is a desirable one, but at times may be something of a pretense. In crisis situations, such as outlined above, it is a contract developed under threat – present threat that without it admission will be withheld; future threat that deviation will break the contract terms and therefore subject the child to sanctions (Hobbs 1975). The child is the focal point for potential three-way blackmail by the parents, the program, and himself. He has been placed in a situation against which he has mechanisms of appeal which can only worsen his lot. He cannot protest to an outside authority, only to his parents who, for their own reasons, are wholly or partly agents of his being there. If he objects by behavior or in words, he can have sanctions applied to him in the name of treatment. He now has to deal not only with the problems he brought but the problems created by the rules of the institution (Goldstein, Freud and Solnit 1973). If he walks out, he can be brought back or lose his opportunity for participation in a program. What more involuntary commitment can there be than where the only authorities to which appeal can be made are those who rule on the validity of the appeal against them?

At the other end of the process – the point of exit – once again the rights are obscured (Juvenile Court Digest 1976). The community from which he came may be more than reluctant to have him re-enter (Goldstein, Freud and Solnit 1973). His choice of alternatives may or may not be heard (Wittenberg 1976) (Hobbs 1975). The agency, be it family or social, often declines to take responsibility on discharge, and other alternatives have to be arranged (Goldstein, Freud, and Solnit 1973) (Holt 1974) (Juvenile Court Digest 1976). While in care, in this quasi-involuntary status, the child or adolescent can be subjected, again for his own good, to a number of potentially arbitrary interventions that may contravene his rights. Frequently, particularly in smaller settings, there is a unitary treatment philosophy, and children fit into this or are in trouble or excluded. Few, except the very large programs, have either professional or resource potential to tailor individual programs to individual needs of children. Medication can and is being used without securing the child's consent, despite considerable evidence that involving the child increases the likelihood of therapeutic effect. The purpose in mentioning these problems is not to criticize or to compound the difficulties of those who work in residential treatment. Heaven knows these are already sufficiently wearying and troublesome. It is, however, to pinpoint the issues that have been identified by some groups, and the partial justification for these. It is also to indicate a concern that externally imposed remedies may make the present situation very much worse. Thus a recent proposal for safeguarding a child's rights within residential programs would require the reading to the child of his rights to disagree, to appeal, the process of appeal, possibility of legal representation and so on. One cannot disagree with the sentiment; but to provide, particularly to the manipulative adolescent, what can only sound like a series of adversarial opportunities may protect his rights but will certainly impede the process of his engagement in a treatment program. This right, incidentally, would have applied to any child over the age of 12 and could well, in practice, lead to extensive legal intervention, and enormous time consumed in preparing reports and defending situations.

The sum total of this and other proposals are being seen by people in residential treatment as almost identifying them as those from whom the child requires the greatest protection. The highly legalistic approach may improve the standard of paperwork; it is certainly not going to improve the availability or dedication of those who work on behalf of the children.

A similar set of standards which would have applied to residential and to foster situations forbids corporal punishment including:

(I) Striking a child, directly or with any physical object.
(II) Shaking, shoving, spanking or other forms of aggressive physical contact.
(III) Punishment of a child by another child or group of children condoned by, or at the instigation of staff.
(IV) Requiring or forcing the child to take an uncomfortable position such as squatting, bending or standing against a wall.
(V) Requiring or forcing the child to repeat physical movements.
(A) Harsh, humiliating, belittling or degrading responses of any form, including verbal, emotional and physical.
(B) Deprivation of what the child is entitled to, or what is necessary for proper development, care or treatment, including but not limited to:
(i) Family visits.
(ii) Food, shelter, clothing or bedding.
(iii) Extensive withholding of emotional response or stimulation.
(iv) Placing or keeping a child in a locked room.
(v) Requiring the child to maintain silent for long periods of time.
(vi) Mechanical or excessive physical restraint.
(vii) Exclusion of the child from entry to the residence.
(viii) Assignment of unduly physically strenuous or harsh work.
(ix) Prolonged confinement to bed.

(Ministry of Community & Social Services Children's Services Division 1978).

These are in fact very close to proposed or accepted legal standards in Sweden. Even there, there is concern for the legal interpretation and enforcement of something as subjective as negative psychological sanction.

These proposals, however, highlight the problem. Such things should not exist. However, people are human and who among us as parent as well as in other roles has not felt like or indeed has occasionally applied a punctuative swat to the rear end of a kid who is cruising in lack of controls? Can we afford to set a standard which is so high that all of us inevitably could be held to be guilty somewhere along the line? Indeed, in response to these proposed changes a group of foster parents cogently stated the problem the changes would present. Parents would have the freedom to bring up their own children in one way, while required to behave at times in a different and artificial manner with the foster children. While the purpose of the overall document of which this was a segment was 'normalization of children's experiences', the proposed standards left very little that would not contravene legislation other than saying, 'Please, would you be kind enough to stop doing this'. This is an approach which the foster parents suggested, and one could only agree, may work some but not all of the time, with some but not with all children, and which is clearly impossible for anyone to implement unless they have the patience of Job.

There is no doubt that in the fields of human service the right of the child to be heard and, where appropriate, to participate has not been honoured as much as it could be. Professionals have known all too well what the children needed. There have been abuses. The proposed correction of these abuses, however, comes often from people who have had no experience of dealing in these situations and threatens to encumber the system in a bureaucratic tangle and eventually to impede or discourage a caring intervention. The staff will spend more time protecting themselves. The challenge is for the institutions of society, both small and large, to be continually attentive and internally vigilant to obviate the necessity for external review of every minutia. It is undoubtedly necessary to recognize that society, particularly when it underwrites the cost, is going to demand a greater voice in the way activities are conducted. To ignore this is to do so at one's peril. Indeed the pressure created by documents that I have cited has already led to substantial improvement and upgrading of procedures.

Neither the legal nor the service systems are the sole protectors of children's rights; neither have all virtue on their side. An adversarial system may keep many people employed and allow fewer children to be treated, while the present creative tension, hopefully, can allow a greater respect for, attention to, and safeguarding of the legal and the ethical rights to which children should be entitled.

Vice-Chairman,
Dept. of Psychiatry,
University of Toronto,
Psychiatrist-in-Chief,
Hospital for Sick Children,
Toronto, Ontario, Canada

REFERENCES

Aries, P.
1970 Centuries of Childhood. A. A. Knopf, New York.
Bremner, P. H., Ed.
1971 Children and Youth in America. Harvard U. Press., Mass.
Celdic
1970 One Million Children. L. Crainford, Pub., Toronto.
Time Magazine
1972 Children's Rights: The Latest Crusade. Dec. 25.
Central Toronto Youth Services
1975 Control Problems and Alternatives to Section 8, Ontario Training Schools Act. Toronto.

Cornfield, P. H.
1975 Emancipation by Eviction: The Problem of Domestic Pushout. The Family Law Reporter, Vol. 1, No. 12: 4021–4028.
Despert, J. L.
1965 The Emotionally Disturbed Child – Then and Now. Vantage Press, N. Y.
Fox, S. J.
1974 The Reform of Juvenile Justice: The Child's Right to Punishment. Juvenile Justice, August, pgs. 2–9.
Fraser, P. G.
1975 The Pediatric Bill of Rights. South Texas Law Journal, Vol. 16, No. 3, pgs. 245–308.
Goldstein, J., Freud, A., and Solnit, A. J.
1973 Beyond the Best Interests of the Child. Free Press, New York.
Guttman, F. M.
1974 On Withholding Treatment. Canadian Medical Association Journal. Vol. 111, pgs. 520–521.
Hobbs, N.
1975 The Futures of Children. Jossey-Pass, Pub., Washington.
Holt, J.
1974 Escape from Childhood: The Needs and Rights of Children. E. P. Dutton and Co., Inc., New York.
Joint Commission on Mental Health of Children
1970 Crisis in Child Mental Health: Challenge for the 1970's. Harper and Row, New York.
Kittrie, N. N.
1971 The Right to be Different. Johns Hopkins Press, Baltimore.
Canadian Mental Health Association (Quebec) Montreal
1974 The Legal Rights of Children.
Lourie, N. V., and Lourie, B. P.
1970 A Non-Categorial Approach to Treatment Programs for Children and Youth. Delivery of Services. Amer. J. Orthopsychiat., Vol. 40, No. 4, July, pgs. 684–693.
Marker, G., and Friedman, P. R.
1973 Rethinking Children's Rights. Children Today, November-December, pgs. 8–11.
Juvenile Court Digest
1976 Mental Commitment of Children. April, pgs. 244–248.
Noltf, M. G.
1976 Are Students 'Persons' Under the Constitution? Goss V. Lopez Implies as Much. Law in American Society – Journal of the National Centre for Law – Focused Education, Vol. 5, No. 1, pgs. 9–15.
Rae-Grant, N. I.
1974 Some Thoughts on Classification, Confusion, Complexity, and Competence in Child Psychiatry. Presented at the 8th Congress of International Associations for Child Psychiatry and the Allied Professions – Philadelphia, August 1.
Rae-Grant, N. I.
1971 The Treatment of Casualties or Causes – An Urgent Question for Child Mental Health – Presented at the American Orthopsychiatry Meeting, Washington, March.
Rae-Grant, Q., and Moffat, P. J.
1971 Children in Canada/Residential Care. Canadian Mental Health Association, Toronto.
Rafferty, F. T.
1964 Symptoms and Process in the Multi-Disciplined Community. Amer. J. Orthopsychiat., Vol. 34, pgs. 569–574.

Redl, F.
1962 Crisis in the Children's Field. Amer. J. Orthopsychiat., Vol. 32 pgs. 759–780.
Harvard Ed. Rev.,
1973 The Rights of Children. Special Issue, Vol. 43–4.
Russell, A. H. The Emancipation of Children. (Unpublished).
The Solicitor General's Committee
1975 Young Persons in Conflict with the Law. Iri-Graphic, Pub., Ottawa.
Sowell, T.
1976 A Black 'Conservative' Dissents. New York Times Magazine, August 8, pgs. 14–16.
State of New York Youth Commission
Children's Bill of Rights.
Hospital and Community Psychiatry
1975 The State of the Child: Highlights from the 52nd Annual Meeting of the American Orthopsychiatric Association. Vol. 26, No. 8, August, pgs. 518–527.
Wittenberg, C. K.
1976 Children's Rights Issues Debated at Annual Meeting. Psychiatric News, Vol. XI, No. 13, pgs. 25–26.
Werry, J., Minde, K., Guzman, A., Weiss, G., Dogan, K. and Hoy, E.
1972 Studies on the Hyperactive Child. VII: Neurological Status Compared with Neurotic and Normal Children. American Journal of Orthopsychiatry 42: 441–451.
Ministry of Community and Social Services, Children's Services Division, Toronto
1978 Children's Residential Care Facilities: Proposed Standards and Guidelines. September.

SECTION FOUR

ISSUES WITH THERAPEUTIC IMPLICATIONS

INTRODUCTION

No work on mental health has credibility which does not at least attempt to forge out of accumulative and accumulating work new pathways to influencing factors which bear on health improvement. It is helpful to review, relearn and rediscover, but ultimately we must face the formidable task of transcending the bounds of previous knowledge. This section is devoted to papers by visionary leaders in mental health who struggle with the task of translating what is known and refining research techniques into effecting change in the mental health systems of nations.

Berner emphasizes that little can be done preventively without sound scientific research. Knowledge alone is insufficient for the proper development of intervention programs. Berner reviews problems of research related to 'case' definitions, validity, and the sensitivity and specificity of the measuring instruments. In addition, he points out the urgent need for an internationally acceptable classification of mental disorders. Without such classification it is difficult to define an individual case of mental illness. Even more difficult is the identification of a case within a system of interactions such as the family.

And yet much progress has been made in delineating the subtle interactions which bear on the emotional health of families. Disturbed communication in families, verbal and non-verbal, holds promise for future research. Notwithstanding the obstacles presented by retrospective studies, difficulties in securing a control population, and the mobility of families, Berner feels that certain research strategies can be developed, rationalized, and brought to bear on preventive measures.

Pardes, in a comprehensive view of initiatives for the new decade, emphasizes, also, the need for more refined diagnostic systems and improved data bases to allow for systematic and definitive studies. Although the focus is on developments in the USA, the principles outlined are widely applicable. Pardes discusses broadening people's access, particularly underserviced populations, to mental health services. He identifies these populations and suggests changes to allow greater access, including fiscal re-arrangements. While expanding access, Pardes suggests delineating more precisely the purview of mental health and recognizing what we can or cannot do. He anticipates a greater role for the mental health sector in linkage with the general health sector where the majority of people are served. Concurrently mental illness must be further destigmatized in order for people to seek psychiatric and psychological assistance.

The role of psychological factors in various diseases has been well enough established to encourage the development of preventive programs and Pardes

S. H. Fine, R. Krell, and Tsung-yi Lin (Eds.), 'Today's Priorities in Mental Health' 109–110.

states increased attention will now be paid toward prevention of psychiatric disorders. Research will focus on issues pertaining to children and families where early intervention will prove useful.

In the final paper, Sartorius points out that not only are psychological development and mental health still low on the priority list of many countries, the idea still prevails that the health of children can be improved by dealing with physical disease first and later with their development. This motion perpetuates a chronic obstacle to the development of an attitude that the health of children and their overall development is the priority, not simply the elimination of one or another disease. Sartorius dramatically emphasizes the absence of services to children. Many of the one hundred million children in developing countries suffering from mental disorders are unknown to the health care system.

What is particularly disconcerting is that effective measures for the prevention and treatment of mental disorders in childhood is, in the broadest sense, available. Sartorius states that a vast proportion of these disorders could be eliminated at a cost that most countries can afford. He cites the areas for intervention and treatment; among them drug treatment for epilepsy at a cost of one dollar per child per year, or glasses to correct vision at a cost of sixty cents.

Sartorius faults increasingly poor communication between agencies and social sectors, the withholding of simple technology, the obscuring of simple information through jargon, the growth of bureaucracies, scarce resources, and the difficulties inherent in changing attitudes of the public, the decision-makers and of professionals.

New strategies of health care are difficult to implement in the face of such massive obstacles. And yet there is hope that the gradual re-emphasis on the self-reliance of people and communities will ensure their obtaining primary health care. It is against a background of self-reliance, technical co-operation and a selection of priorities that WHO and UNICEF have elaborated a policy concerning the mental health and psychosocial development of children. The proposals set out can be turned from policy into reality. Whether or not this happens depends on people like ourselves and our determination to make it happen.

ROBERT KRELL, M. D.

Prof. Dr. PETER BERNER (Austria)

MENTAL HEALTH FOR CHILDREN AND FAMILIES: IMMEDIATE RESEARCH NEEDS

During the plenary sessions and workshops we reviewed the essential aspects of the mental health of children and families. The previous discussions have demonstrated the host of factors thought to have some influence on the mental health of the child or on the future adult. The importance of these factors is seldom demonstrable scientifically. To prove or disprove hypotheses concerning these factors remains a task for the future and must become the subject of exact scientific research. Until such proof is demonstrated, the preventive measures which are our central preoccupation remain an uncertain undertaking. It is the aim of this paper to outline the problems which urgently require research.

All prevention must be based on increased etiological and pathogenetic knowledge. For the time being our etiopathogenetic theories – especially with regard to harmful social influences – are still very incomplete and are based more often on suppositions than on proven facts. That is why any preventive measures deduced from these suppositions cannot yet acquire the status of a well-established strategy. This observation is concerned in the first place with primary prevention but it is applicable as well to a certain degree, to secondary and tertiary prevention. I will limit myself to sketching several problems that research must confront and resolve in order to achieve reliable results in determining the importance of the environmental influences on the origin and the progress of psychological disorders.

1. THE DEPENDENT VARIABLE IN PSYCHIATRIC RESEARCH

Traditional psychiatry concentrates on individual cases and therefore each is defined as precisely as possible. Social psychiatry, on the other hand, is concerned with the 'problem' which occurs in a social system disturbance where the 'case' is only one member of a system. We shall therefore first discuss the difficulties which we encounter in defining cases, and then we shall look at the obstacles we meet when we try to grasp the 'problems' of the family.

(a) *Definition of 'Cases'*

No serious etiopathogenic research can proceed without a precise definition of the cases which are the objects of study. To this end it is necessary to find indicators of the health or illness of the individual. These indicators are generally drawn from screening instruments. Among these are Langner's 22-item question-

S. H. Fine, R. Krell, and Tsung-yi Lin (Eds.), 'Today's Priorities in Mental Health' 111–117.

naire (1962) and its derivatives, which are generally used as a self-evaluation scale. More elaborate methods include Beck's questionnaire and similar scales and finally, scales which the psychiatrist completes on the basis of clinical interviews, such as Hamilton's scale (1960), the 'Present State Examination' (PSE, Wing *et al.*, 1974) or the AMDP system (1979).

Most of these instruments lend themselves as well to a qualitative evaluation of particular psychopathological phenomena. Another type of evaluation which is often applied consists of formulating certain overall scores, which are taken as quantitative indicators of the degree of psychopathology present in the individual being examined. The essential problems posed by these indicators of individual mental health (or illness) are those of validity, sensitivity, and specificity of the instrument used.

Let us look first at the problem of validity. The instruments from which the indicator is taken have in general been validated by psychiatrists who, based on their clinical judgment, have declared whether or not a particular individual was a case. Differences of opinion still hold sway in our discipline in the matter of diagnostic classification on the one hand and of quantitative evaluation of phenomena on the other (the latter can be very important for identifying indicators). These differences mean that we have to be very circumspect in the conclusions to be drawn from these indicators, which are based on the calculation of overall levels.

In cases where validation does not pose a problem, namely when there is a clear consensus on the definition of cases and on the quantification of symptoms (a very rare situation), the sensitivity and specificity of the instrument must still be tested.

Sensitivity is measured by determining the ratio of persons identified as 'cases' by the screening instrument to the total number of actual cases. Specificity, on the other hand, is evaluated by comparing the percentage of people correctly identified as 'negative' by the instrument to the total number of truly negative people.

But even if we use well-validated instruments whose sensitivity and specificity have been found to be satisfactory, we must never forget that the use of overall levels always involves some loss of information, which can distract our attention from the distinction between primary and secondary, or essential and occasional symptoms. That is why, in epidemiological research serving as a basis for the development of preventive strategies, individual indicators can only be used as 'screening instruments' in the strict sense of the word. To ensure greater scientific rigor, we must require all those persons identified by the indicator to undergo a supplementary examination which would be more sophisticated and more detailed than that carried out by the screening instrument.

This requirement is not fulfilled in most clinical and epidemiological research programs. Generally we are content to establish general diagnoses such as schizophrenia or neurosis, perhaps adding an overall estimate of psychopathology as determined by the screening instrument. Many sociological studies do not even go that far, speaking only of 'mental illness'.

But if we start with a general notion of mental illness, we must first attempt to define mental health. In sociological works, such definitions generally refer to ideal norms which have not proved to be of practical use to research. Although we cannot here examine the problem of norms at length, we must nevertheless mention that in any discussion of mental health or illness four types of norms should be defined: the statistical norm, the ideal norm, the functional norm and the observer's subjective norm. The first two are objective, or mathematical norms, which are based on values applicable to all or at least by the majority of the population in question. The latter two are subjective norms.

For the purposes of research we can define mental health only in a negative way – the absence of mental illness. But we can demonstrate that we should, according to the norms to which we are referring and the data we are using, make three definitions of mental illness: the subjective notion of mental illness; the medical notion; and one defined with reference to the premorbid personality. The concept of mental illness is consequently so diverse that it is not applicable as such. The dividing line between unhappiness and illness, for example, cannot be precisely pinpointed by a simple reference to some 'psychological disorder'. If we wish to arrive at pertinent conclusions, we must refer to subtypes of mental disorders or to well-defined syndromes which will vary according to the phenomena we undertake to study. Psychiatry has not yet developed a classification of mental disorders according to syndromes which is acceptable to large groups of researchers. The development of such an internationally acceptable instrument seems to be an urgent task for any etiopathogenetic research.

This is all the more necessary as social systems are 'open systems' which are characterized by the principle of equifinality. This principle stipulates that open systems can result in a state which is independent of time and of the initial state, and which is caused only by the parameters of the system. In psychopathology this means that extremely varied original situations and temporal influences often produce the same syndromes, with the result that research must at the outset be oriented toward the syndrome so that we can detect what factors might play a role in the development of such psychopathological groupings. The phenomenon of equifinality is certainly also responsible for the fact that abnormal behaviour patterns which are even more complex than the syndrome and might be called 'Behaviours', (alcoholism or a suicidal tendency), are often very valuable indicators of those areas in which a social system is functioning well or badly.

(b) *Establishment of Cases*

The validity of the results of any sociological and psychiatric research project depends to a large extent on the selection of cases. According to the time at which mental illness is established, a distinction must be made between prevalence and incidence. Prevalence consists of the total number of psychological disorders existing on a specific day. Incidence, on the other hand, consists of new cases appearing over a specific period of time. When we actually count all the cases in a specific population, we speak of 'true' prevalence or incidence. But if we count, as is often the case with official statistics, only illnesses being treated, we must speak of 'treatment prevalence or incidence'. Each statement about frequency must specify its references, or else no conclusion is possible: etiological conclusions must be based on true incidence, whereas for purposes of planning it might be sufficient to use only treatment prevalence. Watts (1966) used the image of the iceberg to illustrate the differences between these points of reference: only a small part of the iceberg of the number of cases of depression is above the surface of social visibility and is submitted to treatment. The majority of cases of depression go undetected. Treatment prevalence thus cannot in any case lead to conclusions about causality on the social level. If a causal factor is itself a criterion of selection for assigning a patient to an institution, the use of treatment prevalence can be the cause of serious errors.

(c) *The Family as a 'Problem'*

If the definition of the individual case proves to be difficult, and we know that it is, the problem becomes still more complicated when the 'case' is a system of interactions. The family is such a system if we define system as an organization characterized by the stability of its variables and staying within certain limits. The limits are maintained by 'family homeostasis', namely the tendency to accept outside influences and to modify them internally towards equilibrium. A family's ability to do this can constitute a unit of measurement for the health of the family. Some family systems are able to withstand and to absorb some of fate's cruelest blows while others cannot even manage to handle small crises. A most important task for research into family mental health is to operationalize, objectify and quantify this function of assimilating and solving problems.

Although we may still be far from completing the study of these mechanisms we have nevertheless made some progress in the direction of outlining certain specific anomalies in the family system. Early research studied the relationships between disturbances in the family and certain forms of mental illness. These studies were limited to the observation of facts which were easy to apprehend, such as early loss of parents. Current research is now concentrating more on the subtle styles of communication within families. This change is due to the fact that research aiming to establish simple relationships such as the effect of parental loss, or else remaining relatively imprecise with studies such as those on the broken home, has not arrived at any conclusive results. But it is obvious that the more subtle are the interactions under study, the more difficult it becomes to define them. This is why many research workers have not yet succeeded in operationalizing them for use in systematic studies. Many of these very interesting efforts unfortunately still remain at the stage of anecdotal description. However, it would seem that research in the areas of verbal and nonverbal communication within the family opens a fruitful field for future research. Let us mention a few examples. Lidz (1967, 1968) has described two types of marriage which, according to him, occur between the parents of schizophrenics, the skewed and the schismatic family. Another example is the observations of Singer and Wynne (1966) who have described forms of abnormal communication in terms of pseudo-reciprocity and pseudo-hostility, as well as of amorphous and fragmented communication. Although attempts to verify this research have not really succeeded in consolidating the theory of the specificity of schizophrenia, these descriptions nevertheless remain the basis for future research into the disturbed communication within families. The urgent task for research in the area of these communication problems again seems to be the operationalization of the various modes of interaction. We need validated instruments which will make possible large-scale comparisons based on representative populations.

2. INDEPENDENT VARIABLES

The reliability and validity of in_ependent variables in sociopsychiatric research is still very slight. The social influences and situations which these variables represent, such as class or social status, or disturbing events, are far from being defined precisely enough to be used as a basis for solid research. Nevertheless, we must admit that in this area, too, there are great efforts being made to remedy the situation. One example is research into the events of life which may prove to be responsible for psychiatric problems. This research effort has developed reliable instruments such as the 'Life Event Schedule' (Brown, 1974), but much work remains to be done to construct instruments which will allow the satisfactory evaluation of the influence of social factors on mental health and illness.

3. SUMMARY OF IMMEDIATE TASKS FOR RESEARCH

Research into the psychological and social causes of mental disorders and the effectiveness of preventive measures has met with some formidable problems. These concerns especially influence the individual during childhood, while he is with his family. Many mental disorders do not show up until later life, and then it is very difficult to find out to what degree the influence which one underwent during childhood really played a role. Devising measures on the basis of adult population and deriving preventive measures intended for childhood remains an intimidating undertaking. The period of time which elapses between the application of these measures and their effect is often too long to allow us to make convincing conclusions. This is due, on the one hand, to the fact that later influences may be responsible for the appearance or non-appearance of a mental illness, and on the other hand, to the fact that it is extremely difficult to follow a defined population over long periods, especially in societies with a high degree of mobility. Moreover, it is not easy to set up control groups in the area of prevention. This explains why hypotheses about etiopathogenetic factors are often based on retrospective studies which contain many errors. Finally, it is also difficult to isolate certain singular factors which could be responsible for a favorable or unfavorable psychological development. It remains problematical to plan research projects based on specific events such as life-events or even evaluations of family interactions.

But in spite of these difficulties, certain research strategies could be developed which could reduce these obstacles. The development of such strategies is of great importance in opening up possibilities for effective action in the field of prevention. The tasks concerned with research planning must take into account the following points:

(a) That a good definition and establishment of cases be linked to an operationalization of the various modes of family interaction.
(b) That the populations being examined be truly representative.
(c) That independent variables be operationalized more effectively and their relationship with 'cases' and well-defined 'problems' be shown.
(d) That prospective studies must be undertaken involving a long period of observation with the opportunity of frequent intermediate evaluations.

This conference has highlighted the enormous importance of a successful childhood for the mental health of the individual and of society. There is much information which demonstrates in what areas positive or negative influences might have effect, but most hypotheses must still be proved or disproved in order to achieve stronger planning for preventive measures. Our knowledge is still in a state of development. We must bring order to this theoretical and practical material in order to develop strategies for prevention whose efficiency and whose consequences can be constantly monitored and improved.

Algemeines Krankenhaus der Stadt Wien,
Psychiatrische Universitätsklinik,
Vienna, Austria

REFERENCES

A.M.D.P. (Arbeitsgemeinschaft für Methodik und Dokumentation in der Psychiatrie): Das A.M.D.P.-System
1979 Manual zur Dokumentation psychiatrischer Befunde. Springer Verlag, Berlin-Heidelberg-New York.

Beck, A. *et al.*
1961 An inventory for measuring depression. Arch. Gen. Psychiat. 4 pp 561–571.

Brown, G. W.
1974 Meaning, Measurement and Stress of Life Events. In: Dohrenwend, B.S., B. P. Dohrenwend (Eds.): Stressful Life Events: Their Nature and Effects. John Wiley, New York.

Hamilton, M.
1960 A rating scale for depression. J. Neurol. Neurosurg. Psychiat. 23 pp. 36–62.

Langner, T. S.
1962 A twenty-two-item screening score of psychiatric symptoms indicating impairment. J. Hlth. Hum. Behav. 3 pp 269–276.

Lidz, T.
1967 The family, personality development and schizophrenia. In: The origins of schizophrenia, Excerpta Medica International Congress Series Nr. 151.

Lidz, T.
1968 The family, language and the transmission of schizophrenia. In: The Transmission of Schizophrenia, Ed. Rosenthal, D., S. Kety, Oxford.

Singer, M. T., L. C. Wynne
1966 Communication styles in parents of normal neurotics and schizophrenics. Psychiat. Res. Rep. 20 pp 25–38.

Wing, J. K., J. E. Cooper, N. Sartorius
1974 The Measurement and Classification of Psychiatric Symptoms. Cambridge University Press, London.

Watts, C. A. H.
1966 Depressive Disorders in the Community. John Wright & Sons, Bristol.

HERBERT PARDES, M. D. (U.S.A.)

MENTAL HEALTH INITIATIVES FOR THE EIGHTIES

INTRODUCTION

I am delighted to have this opportunity to be here and to participate in this splendid 1979 World Congress on Mental Health. In a world shrunk by modern communications and mutual concerns, it becomes increasingly important that we who work in the mental health field in all areas of the world come together to pool our knowledge and, equally importantly, to share our perspectives. In doing so, we benefit ourselves, our programs, and the individuals that each of us serve.

The 1979 World Congress occurs at a particularly salutary time for mental health programs in the United States. The deep and genuine interest of President Carter and First Lady Rosalyn Carter in the mental health needs of our country was evidenced by the formation, in 1977, of a President's Commission on Mental Health. Mrs. Carter, who served as Honorary Chairperson of the Commission, was pivotal in gaining the broad base of public and professional support necessary to conduct a first-class assessment of the state-of-the-field. She has shown, moreover, great expertise in understanding the substance of mental health issues in the United States, thus assuring that the Report of the Commission to the President will serve as a blueprint for our national health programs in future years.

Since the Report was submitted to the President in April 1978, we at the National Institute of Mental Health with our colleagues in the U.S. Department of Health, Education, and Welfare, have used the Report as a guidepost in planning the future directions of our programs. Over the past year, we have worked intensively to make operational many of the hundred-some recommendations of the President's Commission. Acknowledging that effort, today I would like to outline for you several of the major themes that will be emerging in the U.S. mental health programs over the next 10 to 15 years.

INCREASED RIGOR IN DIAGNOSES AND DATA

A fundamental theme that will be apparent in all facets of our mental health endeavor will involve attempts to secure more refined diagnostic systems, improved data bases, and more clearly documented rationales for our mental health programs. Too often in the past, our diagnostic systems have suffered from a lack of replicability, an inability to evoke broad concensus, and considerable ambiguity. Ambiguity is seen in the criteria for diagnoses as well as in diagnoses *per se*. Contributing to what often may be perceived as a rather chaotic situation with respect to diagnosis have been the countless theories –

S. H. Fine, R. Krell, and Tsung-yi Lin (Eds.), 'Today's Priorities in Mental Health' 119–127.

found in all dimensions of the mental health enterprise, but perhaps most frequently in treatment – that are supported primarily through the fervor and conviction of a few individuals rather than through systematic and definitive studies, rationales, and analyses of data. Today, mental health scientists have unprecedented capabilities to accumulate and rigorously analyze data. I believe that in the future, the mental health system will place greater emphasis on such analyses, both in clinical and administrative spheres, than it has in the past.

ACCESS TO MENTAL HEALTH SERVICES

A second major theme of the President's Commission suggesting a need for increased emphasis within our national mental health program is that of broad access to mental health services. Over the past twenty years we have made great progress in this area. In 1955, there were 1.7 million episodes of care in mental health facilities in the U.S. In 1975, there were 6.9 million episodes of care. During that time, the settings in which people received mental health care dramatically reversed: in 1955, approximately 77 percent of people receiving mental health services did so as inpatients; in 1975, that pattern reversed, with 76 percent of persons receiving outpatient mental health services and only 24 percent treated as inpatients.

Despite these gains, one of the most critical issues identified by the Commision involved the needs of special populations that are presently unserved or underserved by the mental health system. Inadequate service may stem from a number of causes. Many individuals, for example, are physically isolated from the system, be they in sparsely populated rural expanses or in densely populated central metropolitan areas. For other individuals of certain racial and cultural backgrounds, language or cultural traditions may serve as obstacles to mental health care. Age can limit access, particularly for the very old and the very young, reflecting shortages in our country of such specialists as geriatric and child mental health professionals. Economics and financing patterns also block access to mental health care. In the United States, approximately 187 million persons, or some 89 percent of the civilian, non-institutionalized population were covered by public or private health insurance plans or programs in 1975. However, only an approximate 63 percent of the civilian population are covered for inpatient mental health care, while even fewer – 38 percent – have outpatient mental health benefits which often are quite limited. Not only do reimbursement policies frequently discriminate against mental illness, but many people simply cannot afford to obtain what may be the most appropriate service for their particular need.

One other population of persons has gained increasing recognition in the United States as lacking access to needed comprehensive mental health services – the chronically mentally ill. Historically, variations in the treatment and management of chronic patients have reflected complex social, economic, philosophic, and therapeutic considerations. At one point, chronic patients were relegated to hospitals cut off from the mainstream of society, well out of the public eye. More recently, given a critical look at the nature of these hospitals and their effects on patients, attempts have been made to deinstitutionalize patients rapidly. However, various observers have noted that deinstitutionalization frequently is simply a process of 'dehospitalization': i.e., patients may be moved from hospitals to other institutions such as nursing homes that offer little increased opportunity to interact in communities.

In the face of these imbalances, there is increasing conviction and determination in the U.S. that mental health services should be made truly accessible to all persons. Means of assuring improved accessibility will require adjustments in a number of areas, including the financing patterns for mental health care, policies that influence the training and education of mental health professionals, and continuity and linkage of mental health with other health and human service programs.

With regard to chronic patients, proper access requires that we attend to such individuals wherever they are, and that we are not single-mindedly preoccupied with the notion that institutions are bad or good unto themselves. Rather, institutions of various types must be made optimally responsive to patients' needs. Two years ago, the National Institute of Mental Health, (NIMH) launched its Community Support Program to work particularly with chronic patients. The aim of this program is to assure that a variety of services and support systems needed by chronic patients to function optimally outside a mental institution are made available to them. Facets of the program also are directed toward the needs of patients who remain in hospitals. One of the key features of the Community Support Program is the assignment of responsibility for monitoring individual patients' needs to a particular 'case manager'; every effort is made to assure that patients do not fall between bureaucratic cracks.

Many of the obstacles to service that I have described were identified by the President's Commission on Mental Health, and on the basis of that body's recommendations, we in the federal mental health establishment have developed and proposed new legislation, the Mental Health Systems Act, that is particularly responsive to the needs of underserved populations.

The Mental Health Systems Act is a modification and refinement of the community mental health centers program that was begun in the United States in 1963. The Systems Act proposes a new partnership between the Federal and State governments that is designed to encourage cooperation among public and private providers of mental health services and that will offer increased flexibility in providing community-based mental health services. Various sections of the Act address the needs of chronically mentally ill adults and children, prevention activities, means of strengthening planning for mental health services, and community-based service needs. Unlike the prior legislation that required communities receiving federal funding to establish fully comprehensive programs at the outset, the new Act would allow the funding of services targeted to populations most in need in particular communities. Over the next several months, the Congress will work toward enactment of this proposal into law.

In the context of congressional action, I should note also that President Carter's Administration recently has suggested to the Congress major modifications of the Medicare and Medicaid programs that offer public financial assistance to people in need of mental health care but who lack other sources of financial access. Changes in the Federal programs would improve, for children and elderly persons, both the amount of reimbursement available through these programs and the types of services that would be offered. For example, regulations that currently require the provision of inpatient services would be modified to allow the use of outpatient mental health services where they would be more appropriate to the patients' needs.

THE BOUNDARIES OF MENTAL HEALTH

In addition to the themes of greater rigor and increased accessibility to mental health services, I contend that there will be increasing attempts in future years to delimit more precisely the purview of mental health. During the 1960s, there was a tendency in the United States to attribute to mental health a capability for resolving diverse social as well as psychiatric problems. There was legitimate recognition that economic forces and employment opportunities, the quality of housing and of work, and various other social issues did have an impact on mental health. While recognition of the impact of these multiple forces on an individual's mental health was legitimate, it was less appropriate to assume that mental health programs and institutions should – or could – undertake the responsibility of curing those social conditions.

I would argue that it is appropriate for mental health professionals to identify and, inasmuch as possible, document for appropriate social agencies the impact of their policies on the mental health of society. Moreover, with regard to the mental health needs of specific individuals, it is not only appropriate but important for mental health professionals to direct attention to, if not manipulate, social variables that impact on mental health. Yet in both of these spheres of activity, it is essential that mental health professionals recognize and complement the efforts of those social agencies, government institutions, and other entities that have primary responsibility for social problems *per se*.

LINKAGE WITH THE GENERAL HEALTH SECTOR

Even as mental health is reassessing and more precisely delimiting its domain, the field will simultaneously increase its linkages with the general health care sector. This trend already is becoming noticeable; for a number of years now, the Psychiatry Education Branch of the NIMH has promoted programs of medical student education as well as consultation-liaison efforts with primary care and other medical departments. Recent studies conducted in the United States have shown that some 57 percent of persons seeking help for mental health problems are treated *solely* in the general health care sector. Also, a number of studies now suggest that the inclusion of mental health services within general health care programs serves to reduce the utilization of general health services and also has a substantial impact on the overall cost of the identified health care system. In addition to these benefits of more reduced utilization and possibly reduced cost, the patient obviously receives more appropriate care.

I might note that this general issue is familiar to most physicians who have had the experience of seeing patients with somatic presentations of psychological problems. Such patients often receive help from numerous physicians and clinics until such time as they seek psychiatric or psychological treatment. Subsequently, the utilization of general health services often declines.

Another force that may move the mental health system into closer alignment with the general health system is the recognition that in integrated settings where mental health is linked closely with general health services, patients are more likely to be referred for diagnosis, evaluation or consultation with a mental health specialist than when the mental health system is sequestered.

Finally, given the continuing expansion of our therapeutic arsenal – and the dramatic increases in our understanding of biological and psychopharmacological aspects of mental health – the linkage between mental health and health systems is likely to be even more intensively stimulated.

As I mentioned a moment ago, we at the NIMH have recognized the significance of these issues and trends, and have launched a number of programs to encourage and enhance future developments. We are looking, for example, to place mental health professionals in general health settings. We also are emphasizing the training and educational needs of medical students, primary health care and general health care professionals in psychiatric and behavioral principles. In April of this year, NIMH co-sponsored with the Institute of Medicine of the National Academy of Sciences, a conference regarding the critical linkage of mental health and primary care.

DESTIGMATIZING MENTAL ILLNESS

A somewhat related trend that I believe will emerge increasingly over the next several decades, will involve destigmatization of mental illness and of mental health care. We are seeing this already in the United States. Twenty-five and 30 years ago, many people considered the seeking of psychiatric and psychological assistance as taboo. Today, the phenomenon of people seeking mental health help is much more apparent in literature, radio, television, and film; it is also borne out to a much greater degree in the behavior of the population. In a recent study conducted at the University of Michigan that compared attitudes toward mental health care in 1957 to those in 1976, the researchers found a much greater readiness for people to recognize mental health problems and to seek help for them. They found also a greater tendency of people in the lowest economic sectors to seek mental health care, a behavior formerly more typical of persons in the higher socioeconomic sectors.

These developments should not be taken to suggest that stigma is no longer a problem. I wholeheartedly agree with the President's Commission on Mental Health that it is still a most serious and pervasive problem, and one that warrants the Nation's active response. At the NIMH, we are working on a number of strategies that would further reduce the problem of stigma. The inclusion of a mental health package in a National Health Insurance scheme introduced recently by President Carter would allow for increased mental health service reimbursements. As services become more broadly available economically, the access will work toward the reduction of their stigmatization.

In other spheres, we admittedly have much to accomplish with regard to promoting the employment of persons with mental health problems, with regard to ensuring appropriate housing, and other basic opportunities that too often are restricted unfairly. However, there are signs that we are making progress. For example, the Department of Health, Education, and Welfare and the Department of Housing and Urban Development are working cooperatively to arrange housing opportunities. Last year, housing in the community was made available to 1000 patients, and this year, we plan to meet the residential needs of an additional 2500 chronically mentally ill patients.

PREVENTION ACTIVITIES

Complementing the trends and directions that I have described thus far will be a much increased emphasis on programs of prevention in the future. Again, this is an issue that was underscored by the President's Commission, and as a result, considerable resources will be programmed into prevention activities.

One aspect of the prevention initiatives relates to my earlier discussion of health and mental health linkages. With the recognition that diverse behavioral issues have an impact on general medical problems, behavioral health and prevention emerges as an issue of broad concern and interest. For example, the role of psychological factors in cardiovascular disease has been studied extensively, and there is a growing consensus that the A–B personality dichotomy constitutes an important factor in the development of coronary artery disease. In such diseases as diabetes, peptic ulcers, hypertension, and asthma, psychological factors have been implicated. A focus on prevention from a behavioral standpoint holds the promise to offer possible amelioration of these and other major medical disorders. With the suggestion of behavioral impact on the immune system, there are even some health scientists who now suggest a possible role for psychological interventions in such illnesses as cancer.

Apart from the role of prevention in non-psychiatric medical illnesses, increased attention will be directed toward its potential *vis-à-vis* psychiatric disorders. Under the major prevention initiatives presently being launched by the National Institute of Mental Health, a number of issues are targeted for increased research. These include:

the impact of disruptive marriages on children and families;

the promotion of parenting capacities in teenage parents;

the identification of risk factors, such that prevention of such major mental disorders as depression among groups thought to be at high risk – for example, social isolates, single parents, and disadvantaged minorities – might become a possibility;

improving emotional, cognitive, and interpersonal competence among school-age children.

In each of these areas and others, we anticipate that early intervention will prove useful in preventing crippling mental and emotional disorders, or at least will have an impact on the intensity of their ultimate presentation.

INCREASING THERAPEUTIC CAPACITIES

A final theme that I would suggest as having a major impact on mental health directions over the next several decades will be that of the increasing breadth and refinement of the therapeutic armamentarium. Thirty years ago, the therapeutic interventions available to the mental health field were relatively narrow, essentially limited to psychoanalysis, long-term psychotherapy, group therapy, and electro-shock therapy. All of these remain important tools today. But in addition, we have seen a tremendous expansion, both in the psychosocial therapies, with the introduction of brief therapy, family therapy, milieu therapy, crisis intervention, and so on, and in the biological therapies, via the major tranquilizers, antidepressants, lithium, and so forth. Ongoing research in the neurosciences, in psychosocial therapeutics, and in other fields promises to further expand current treatment capacities.

I believe that in the future we will see a much greater attention to the specification of which populations and which symptoms call for particular types of therapeutic interventions. Also, the notion of combined treatments, promises to increase the appropriateness of our treatments – both psychosocial and psychopharmacological – for specific conditions.

THE MENTAL HEALTH OF CHILDREN AND FAMILIES

Given the list of emerging themes and directions that I have described, I would like to describe how these relate to our concerns regarding children and family issues in mental health. For some time, child mental health has been of highest priority at the National Institute of Mental Health. Among programs and initiatives that we have recently launched on behalf of childrens' mental health needs are:

1. Initiation of an effort on behalf of seriously disturbed children that

is referred to as the Most-In-Need Program. A primary focus of this program will be to help coordinate the variety of services needed to ensure the greatest support for chronically and seriously disturbed children.

2. An Administration proposal that would require that all States make available ambulatory mental health care services for children and youth. The proposal, is designed to smooth out the uneven availability of services that has been typical from State to State in the United States in the past. It would assure some minimum level of service availability throughout the country.

3. A redirection of the NIMH's basic mental health training policy that would increase the responsiveness of education and training programs to the mental health needs of underserved populations, including children.
   As I mentioned earlier, the President's Commission designated priority populations in the manpower area, and the Commission's recommendations were in keeping with those made by a Manpower Policy Analysis Task Force of the Alcohol, Drug Abuse, and Mental Health Administration. The policy redirection that I referred to will ensure training in child mental health in our basic programs and will result in an increased production of child mental health specialists.

4. Prevention activities that will focus on children and youth include those which I described a moment ago, such as the impact of marital disruption on youth, the impact of the psychotic parent on children, the promotion of parental skills for teenage parents, and mental health education skills for youth.

5. The appointment of a new NIMH Assistant Director for Children and Youth, who is a child psychiatrist, and will coordinate activities throughout the Institute that pertain to children and youth.

6. Initiation, under the proposed new Mental Health Systems Act that I referred to earlier, of a set of special initiatives which would allow mental health services to be developed for a variety of populations with particular needs – one of the most important of these being children.

7. A rather comprehensive look at our overall research program with the aim of enhancing and increasing the amount of research we support in the area of children's mental health. Questions of appropriate diagnosis, appropriate treatments, the understanding of early development and its impact on mental health and illness, and other issues, are of critical importance to the mission of the NIMH.

I have provided this list of child mental health related activities to emphasize our conviction that a focus on children's mental health, with particular attention directed toward the type of early identification and intervention efforts that are typical of prevention efforts, seems a most propitious way of approaching many mental health issues. We anticipate that the next several decades will see an increasing development of knowledge, manpower expertise, and mental health services that focus on children's mental health needs. Clearly part of such a focus would be attention to the mental health needs of families as well. A recognition of the psychological interdependence of people within a given system, and particularly within a family system, is longstanding. However, it has only been within the past 25 years that a focus on family therapy and combined treatment interventions for parents and children have become more prominent in common clinical practice. Also within the fairly recent past, various issues regarding parenting have drawn increasing attention from mental health professionals. These changes, the large number of divorces, as well as the multiple patterns of family life, would seem to mandate more sensitivity and research attention to the mental health aspects of family life.

In this context, I might note that the Administration of our country plans to sponsor, in 1981, a White House Conference on Families. Though the focus of the conference will be broad, you may be interested to know that a 1976 survey indicated that among all U.S. Federal agencies, the NIMH supported the greatest amount of research focusing directly on families, and was second only to the Office of Education in the amount of research supported that indirectly focuses on families. The NIMH is currently preparing a major volume that describes in considerable detail approximately forty of our research projects pertinent to the mental health of families; it will be published in conjunction with the White House Conference.

In summary, as I attempt to look toward the future, I see the mental health system becoming more rigorous and more clearly supported by data rather than by fervor. I see the system increasingly accessible to all populations, more delimited in its scope, and, at the same time, more closely linked to general health concerns. I foresee a stronger emphasis on prevention, the development of a broader and more effective therapeutic armamentarium, and increasing attentiveness to the mental health needs of children and families. The prognosis that stems from all these considerations is an exciting era with many opportunities for those who are interested in all facets of mental health. As we work to capitalize on the potentials for advance in each of these areas, and thereby to develop an increasingly refined and sensitive mental health system, I would urge each of us to work as cooperatively as possible on an international basis. If we successfully share our knowledge and our perspectives, we also should have many mutual accomplishments in which to take pride and many patients or would-be patients will feel and function better as a result.

Director,
National Institute of Mental Health,
Rockville, Maryland, U.S.A.

NORMAN SARTORIUS, M.D., Ph.D., F.R.C. Psych. (Switzerland)

THE CHALLENGE OF CHILD MENTAL HEALTH AND DEVELOPMENT: WHO/UNICEF RESPONSE

An old Celtic song tells the story of an apple tree, wind and a gardener. The gardener brings water and tries to protect the young tree; the northern wind whips the sapling and makes it bend. The tree might grow or die: the listener is asked to say which of the three he would like to be – the powerful wind that can break any tree; the gardener who tries to keep the tree alive; or the tree itself, exposed to winds and danger.

The tree, says the listener; because it lives; because it knows danger and tries to best it; because it is grateful and happy when watered and protected; because it is afraid when the wind blows and happy to survive.

At least a billion children in the developing world grow under great stress and in constant danger to their very lives. Those who are to protect and nourish them often have no means or knowledge which would allow them to do so. Some survive and many, unnecessarily, die. Of the survivors many remain scarred, deprived of their chance to live a full life.

The listener to the song decided to be the fragile tree because he wanted to fight, survive, feel happy, grateful or frightened: It was the mental life, the experience of living which he put highly in making his decision, not the mere fact of survival.

Philosophers, decision makers and politicians all agree that the mental health and development of children matters and that it is an essential guarantee for a better tomorrow. And yet, when it comes to action, psychosocial development and mental health are still low on the priority lists of many countries. Undoubtedly, treatment of physical disease is of tremendous importance and will have a significant impact on mental health and development of children: but the idea that it is possible to improve the health of children by first dealing with physical diseases and then later with their mental health and development is dangerous and incorrect. Improved somatic condition is as much a component of health as mental functioning: one cannot be achieved without the other: however, it is the *health* of children and their overall *development* that should have priority over efforts to reduce the prevalence of one or another disease. Children who are malnourished, infested by parasites, sick with a multitude of diseases cannot use their mental potentialities properly: but should we forget that it is the mental life that gives meaning to the existence of a human, we shall create people who are empty, purposeless and emotionally crippled.

But, quite apart from the fact that mental life is an essential component of human existence, mental disorders deserve urgent attention in their own right.

S. H. Fine, R. Krell, and Tsung-yi Lin (Eds.), 'Today's Priorities in Mental Health' 129–133.

Surveys of the general population show that the prevalence of persistent and socially handicapping mental health problems among children aged 3–15 years in developed countries is about 5–15% and more limited data from developing countries suggest a roughly similar rate. These numbers do not include children with mental retardation nor those with diseases such as epilepsy, organic brain syndromes, sensory impairments, and systemic physical diseases; the latter group of diseases often coexists with and aggravates emotional problems, conduct disorders and impairments or delays in the development of normal functions which are among the most frequent mental disorders of childhood (WHO 1977).

If these figures are correct – and they are based on the best available knowledge – then in developing countries alone at least one hundred million children suffer from mental disorders, often complicated by or complicating physical diseases.

Many of these children are unknown to the health care system: but even those who come forward are numerous and usually inappropriately handled. A WHO study demonstrated that up to one-third of all contacts of children with general health care services in an urban slum area are due to mental disorders. In rural areas of Africa and Asia figures were lower but still reaching as much as 10–15% of all contacts with services.

Only one child in four will complete the first six years of school in some Latin American countries and a good proportion of school dropouts could not continue schooling because of (usually unrecognized) mental health problems. Juvenile delinquency, drug taking and alcohol abuse also seem to be growing even among younger children.

These figures assume even more dramatic importance in the light of the fact that effective measures for the prevention and treatment of mental disorders in childhood are now available and that with concerted action a vast proportion of mental disorders in childhood and their consequences in later life could be wiped out at a cost that most countries in the world can easily afford.

Improved maternal and obstetric care could reduce perinatal complications, brain damage and mental health problems associated with it. Better nutrition coupled with appropriate psychosocial stimulation, effective immunization programmes and improved general health care, appropriate accident prevention measures and better care for the chronically handicapped to prevent the occurrence of mental complications are all preventive general health measures that are immediately applicable and of proven efficacy. Social welfare measures – such as the avoidance of unstable and discontinuous patterns of parenting; improvement of day care facilities, hospitals and residential facilities, for example by ensuring continuity of staff taking care of children; review and adjustment of legislation; raising awareness of the psychosocial needs of children and other measures – are all within reach and could have measurable benefits.

Other measures also seem valuable, although definitive knowledge about their efficacy is lacking: here, the addition of evaluative research to planned changes may have immense benefits. Areas in which such research must be undertaken include schooling, the influence of urbanization and industrialization on child health, ways of providing child care in residental institutions and an examination of factors that protect child health in situations which are apparently exposing children to high risk of mental disorder.

The situation is similar in the area of treatment. Evaluative research undertaken in various countries resulted in good evidence about the efficacy of certain measures – such as focussed short term counselling and behavioural methods – which are applicable at primary health care level and at a low cost. Epilepsy is amenable to drug treatment at a low cost and it has been shown that such treatment can be provided at the community level. The yearly supply of medicaments necessary to treat a child with epilepsy can be as low as one US dollar: there are, in sub-Saharan Africa alone, no less than 2 to 3 million children who suffer from this condition and receive little or no treatment. Sensory deficits such as poor vision could be corrected by eyeglasses which cost – pressed from unbreakable plastic – 60 cents US: yet these do not figure on the list for purchases of health services because the importance of sensory stimulation for normal mental development has not been given sufficient prominence.

The optimism and hope which draw strength from the fact that effective and simple methods for the prevention and treatment of disorders in childhood are available and that it is known what could facilitate and foster normal psychosocial development of children of the world must become our main allies in the fight to overcome the multiple constraints which block progress. These constraints include the following:

First, the collaboration and communication among the many agencies and social sectors that should join hands in improving child health is poor and becoming worse. Programmes carried out in educational institutions, institutions which deal with social welfare, and health institutions, compete rather than complement each other. The medical profession, which earlier in this century saw collaboration with teachers as a necessary evil that made immunization campaigns and similar mass health measures easier to implement, has become more and more entrenched and isolated from other sectors, including education. The other relevant professions have also become obsessively concerned with the protection of professional interests, often to the exclusion of considerations of quality and quantity of service they are to render.

Second, the technology which could be made available for use at all levels of health care has been retained in the hands of superspecialists who at best advise other members of their team to treat children nicely, parents wisely and all other professionals suspiciously. How to implement concrete and simple measures that can be taught to a mother, nurse, nursing aid, social worker and many others is often not disclosed; or, when disclosed the action is wrapped in jargon and a cloud of possible dangerous consequences that will ensue unless the specialist is consulted continuously. Parallel to this tendency is the procedure whereby patients with whom progress is slow or difficult to achieve are dumped into facilities or onto professions that have neither resources nor knowledge to provide adequate help.

Third, bureaucracies have, in many places, grown faster than science. They have managed to impose a variety of requirements which sap the strength of the operational part of the apparatus and turn able helpers into inept scribes providing reams of paper which will justify even more paperwork and even less outward-oriented action.

Fourth, health care, on the whole, has become marked by over-reliance on technology and consequent neglect of its human aspects. In the area of child health this tendency is particularly pernicious, not least because children do not choose where they will go when sick and are even less able than adults to offer resistance to unnecessary and abasing treatment.

Fifth, resources are scarce, particularly in developing countries. Facilities are few and badly in need of restoration; there are no staff, no funds and no essential supplies. In most developing countries there is no more than one psychiatrist per two million population; pediatricians are also in short supply; nursing and paramedical staff are far too few. Furthermore, in many countries, there are no posts for those who are qualified.

Sixth, the attitudes of the public, of decision-makers and of professionals are not supportive of new strategies of health care, particularly in the field of mental health. A change of attitudes is difficult to achieve even when all the conditions favouring such a change are fulfilled. In the instance of health care in general and child mental health care in particular, the models of highly developed countries are not always conducive to a new approach. Those who advise and are convinced of the importance of primary health care and other community efforts would have to start at home and undo what they feel should not be started elsewhere.

Seventh, societal and cultural changes have created situations of increased risk to mental health and normal development in many countries. The breakdown of traditional social support systems, including the extended family, replacement of community participation by communal services, information overload and many other facts which, perhaps inevitably, happen on the road to progress, have their side effects. Many of these could be prevented if given sufficient attention in programme development.

Finally, there are demographic changes, such as the increased expectancy of life, in part, resulting from our successes in overcoming some killer diseases of the past. These lead to an increase of numbers of severely disabled children in most countries of the world.

In the presence of these constraints and difficulties, a new strategy of work in the field of health became a necessity. Countries of the world expressed this with more and more clarity and decided, in a series of historic resolutions, that the single most important social goal for them is Health for All by the Year 2000; and that the principal approach to this goal is primary health care.

Primary health care differs from basic health services and from other approaches known to medicine in that it places major emphasis on reliance of people and communities on themselves, on their own strength; in that it requires that social service sectors work together and support each other; and in that it restricts the role of the health sector to those tasks that it knows how to do and can do better than other sectors.

Technical cooperation among countries is the second principal approach to health for all: equitable interdependence and mutual support rather than dependence and charitable aid were put forward as traits of this new relationship.

The third important principle and strategy is the selection of priorities by their social relevance thus reintroducing into health care such public health criteria as prevalence, severity of consequences and out ability to change things.

On this background WHO and UNICEF have recently agreed on their policy concerning mental health and psychosocial development of children (JCHP 1979). This policy reflects principles embedded in primary health care, in socially relevant medicine and in equitable cooperation among countries. It puts emphasis on the education of parents and other community agents so that they can perform their role in facilitating healthy psychosocial development of children; it requires and proposes mechanisms that will make it possible for different social sectors to work together and achieve more with their efforts; it promotes legislative and other social measures that will create the environment in which a child can grow and live; it also makes it imperative to translate the best available knowledge into techniques which health workers can use in their daily work; finally it facilitates cooperation among countries in research, training and provision of facilities and resources for child care.

The implementation of measures which will turn policies into reality depends on governments, professionals, non-governmental organizations and communities. It depends on people like ourselves and our joint determination to work towards a noble social goal: that of making it possible for children of the world not only to survive but also to live, to know why they live and what is happening to them.

Director,
Division of Mental Health,
World Health Organization,
Geneva, Switzerland

REFERENCES

WHO

1977 Child Mental Health and Psychosocial Development, Report of a WHO Expert Committee, Technical Report Series 613, Geneva. ISBN 92–4–120613–6.

United Nations Economic and Social Council

1979 Report of the UNICEF – WHO Joint Commission on Health Policy (JCHP), E/ICEF/L. 1390.

SECTION FIVE

SPECIAL EVENTS

INTRODUCTION

This section is devoted to two special Congress events:

THE YOUTH PANEL

This included eleven young participants from five different countries under the coordination of Drs. Beiser and Cedarbled. They examined five different issues as they affected them personally. These were: the value of schools and education; parent-child relationships; the breakdown of the influence of the extended family; the effects of working mothers; and the relevance of the conference to them. They end with a fitting criticism about not being consulted more when they, the young people, are the subjects of discussion and study. They hope that there will be more collaboration with the youth in future conferences, and this was emphasized by the coordinators.

THE MARY HEMINGWAY REES MEMORIAL LECTURE

This is about the relationship of religion to mental health. Dr. Runions examines the deeper significance of attitudes and values, and how these can affect relationships between mental health professionals and clients. Dr. Runions argues that no one can be completely objective; and, further, that this is not to be decried. We must be hopeful to be helpful; and hope is an attitude.

Religion has given us a theoretical framework and indeed a vocabulary to describe interpersonal relationships: to be salutary these require respect, love and trust, and acceptance of the uniqueness of each individual.

STUART FINE, M.B.

S. H. Fine, R. Krell, and Tsung-yi Lin (Eds.), 'Today's Priorities in Mental Health' 137.

MORTON BEISER, M.D., (Canada), MARTIN GUEST (Canada)
MARIANNE CEDERBLAD, M.D., (Sweden)

THE YOUTH PANEL: A SYMPOSIUM

Dr. Morton Beiser – The young people who constitute our panel have been attending our Congress plenary sessions and some of the workshops. Now it is their turn to speak.

We are going to start with one of the comments of Dr. Spock. He said that the schools do not teach enough about how to live meaningful lives, how to live together in harmony and how to raise children.

WHAT ARE YOUR VIEWS ABOUT SCHOOLS AND EDUCATION

Martin, Canada – Schools teach academic subjects. But within the schools themselves, the most useful and practical experience people get is living with peers and friends. The key education comes not from the classroom but from the experience of living in a mini-society.

Constantine, Greece – I disagree with Martin on one point. First of all we should consider schooling in two dimensions: school in class and school outside of class. If the school system is well-organized, the lessons interesting and the teacher good, you will always learn and what you learn will help you later on in life. Outside of the class you learn from your peer group which provides a model of the society in which you are going to live.

Sandy, USA – The academic subjects are fine for what they do but the teachers lack insight into the problems of adolescents. We all know that adolescence is a very trying time of life. If teachers had more psychological understanding, students would be able to communicate better with the teacher. Many would feel easier about themselves at home as well, providing they felt better understood at school. In the classroom it is extremely important that the teacher be aware not only of learning disabilities but also the various emotional problems which intrude in the life of an adolescent.

Constantine, Greece – In school in Greece you don't have any elective lessons until the last two years. Everything is set down and sometimes it does not seem to make sense. For example, you have to take Ancient Greek for 10 years which doesn't seem very helpful in preparing for life. It seems wasteful.

Martin, Canada – Constantine, you are upset by the 10 years of Ancient Greek. Are you saying that schools should concentrate more on vocational training that is useful only in a practical sense? Should schools not pursue learning for its own sake?

S. H. Fine, R. Krell, and Tsung-yi Lin (Eds.), 'Today's Priorities in Mental Health' 139–143.

Constanine, Greece – You should do that until perhaps Grade 9. By then most students have decided what they want to do with their lives and should be able to take electives in which they have special interest.

Sandy, USA – Constantine says that by the time you are in Grade 9 you have decided what you want to do with your life. I find that not true, at least, in the United States. There are many students who are lost in the educational system and who neither know where to go or what to do. I am very anxious about what is going to happen to me.

Michel, Austria – At the French school in Vienna at about age 15 we may select one of three program sections; a Literature Section, an Economic Section and a Biological and Mathematical Section. I like having such a choice. For example, I may take the Literature Section because in that one has to study more philosophy than in the other sections. This allows a choice of depth and direction.

HOW DO YOUNG PEOPLE SEE THEIR RELATIONSHIP WITH THEIR PARENTS DEVELOPING?

Constantine, Greece – First I should identify myself as a member of a nuclear family. I have very good relations with my parents with whom I communicate well. In a good parent-child relationship what counts most is mutual trust.

Martin, Canada – It is difficult to generalize about such relationships. They are as varied in number as there are parents and children. Those who probably need to talk to their parents most are frequently not capable of it. Their situation deteriorates due to this inability, whereas something may have been done to correct their situation, given better communication.

Judith, Kenya – The key word for parent/child relationships is "understanding". I think that parents should understand their children and vice versa. Without understanding it is hard to consider yourselves as a family.

David, USA – Trust is one of the most important things in a parent/child relationship but in order to secure that trust one has to have total honesty between the parents and the children. Parents do not need to tell children everything but what they do tell them should be truthful.

DO YOU THINK IT IS DESIRABLE TO RETURN TO THE EXTENDED FAMILY?

Sandy, USA – In the USA the extended family is increasingly rare. For example, I know only one aunt on my mother's side and no other family. In the USA families are very mobile and move basically as a nuclear family, consisting of parents and children.

Walid, Kuwait – In our country we still have extended families and find tender emotions and warmth in all its members, including aunts and uncles. The extended family is particularly helpful when a mother works.

Michel, Austria – As far as the extended family is concerned, in the industrialized world, the extended family perhaps no longer has a place because nuclear families are too self-sufficient. Certainly we still have extended families in developing countries but they are likely to disappear. The extended family is important in an agricultural society where you have to rely on manual labor and in a manner of speaking, the extended family offers you workers.

WHAT ARE YOUR PERSONAL EXPERIENCES REGARDING WORKING MOTHERS VERSUS MOTHERS WHO STAY AT HOME?

Martin, Canada – In my opinion it is not good for young children to have a working mother. But at a later age it allows the child greater independence and frees the mother to pursue a career.

Constantine, Greece – It is important for children to not always be with their parents, but I don't think they should be absent all day and available only on weekends. I prefer that mothers work.

Lena, Kuwait – It is alright with me that my mother goes to work. We don't have any specific problems because we are supported by the extended family. I would like her to be with us in the afternoon if that were possible.

Margaret, USA – I have experienced the working mother. Mine is away for three days a week and I think it has made me closer to her because I appreciate her more when she is home. During her absence I spend a lot of time with father so I have more time with each of them. I don't know if I would really want her to stay home and sit around the house because she should lead her life too.

David, USA – Both of my parents work full time and I have never felt that our family was pulled apart, even psychologically separated, because of it. They were home in the evenings, some afternoons and on weekends.

Judith, Kenya – I don't really mind it when my mother works. We have a very good relationship which is not impaired by her working.

FROM WHAT YOU HAVE HEARD AT THE CONFERENCE THIS WEEK DO YOU THINK IT IS OR HAS BEEN OF REAL RELEVANCE TO YOU? DO YOU HAVE SUGGESTIONS FOR FUTURE MEETINGS ABOUT FAMILIES AND CHILDREN?

Martin, Canada – This Congress was supposed to focus on the Year of the Child. In general discussions have been about younger children and we felt that it was necessary to provide an adolescent viewpoint. We might have communicated something the congress participants were not aware of and I think it has been a very good idea to include an adolescent panel.

Sandy, USA – Most of this audience are professionals who have been working with children and adolescents. But being of a different age group, it is probably hard for them to communicate with us. Panels such as this may assist you in better understanding of adolescents and interest you in working with them.

Margaret, USA – I am glad that the congress organizers allowed us to represent ourselves. If you have come to learn about children or adolescents I guess there is no one better to learn it from.

Constanine, Greece – I think that we all agree that the adolescents weren't very well represented at this Congress and that this may be the best way of getting our views across. We need the help in learning to communicate and using those skills to improve our world.

Lena and Walid, Kuwait – Our mother is a participant in the Congress and tells us a great deal about the various topics in the workshops. This is very profitable to us as we have discussed points that pertain to our lives and our relationships with our parents. We are glad to see the attention of parents directed to the needs and welfare of children to secure better mental health. We will be the better for it.

Marianne Cederblad – The situation that we have at this Congress is very typical of how we treat other matters pertaining to children and adolescents in our society. We bring them along and tell them to go and play and not interfere with the very serious matters we must discuss concerning them. We very seldom think of including adolescents as responsible and intelligent people who have valuable experiences and much knowledge to convey. This panel illustrates how our Congress and future Congresses can be enriched by the participation of young people.

Morton Beiser,

Professor of Psychiatry,
University of British Columbia;
Director of Research,
World Health Organization Center for Research and Training in Mental Health,
Vancouver,
British Columbia, Canada.

Marianne Cederblad,

Swedish Association for Mental Health,
Stockholm, Sweden.

PARTICIPANTS

Kristin Carney (USA)
Judith Gachukia (Kenya)
Michel Glaubauf (Austria)
David Gochman (USA)
Alexandra Guest (Canada)
Martin Guest (Canada)
Constantine Lyketsos (Greece)
Alexander 'Sandy' Nadler (USA)
Lena Nassralla (Kuwait)
Walid Nassralla (Kuwait)
Margaret Satersmoen (USA)

(Rev.) J. ERNEST RUNIONS, M.D., F.R.C.P.(C), M.R.C.Psych. (Canada)

The Mary Hemingway Rees Memorial Lecture

FROM HAND TO HAND:

Mental Health, Transmission of Values and Religion

I. INTRODUCTION

The call to examine values in relationship to mental health work arises from many quarters. The work of psychoanalytic theorists; the trenchant observations of the various humanistic psychologies; the vigorous attack of the 'anti-psychiatry' movement; the increasing sophistication of pastoral psychologists; the abuses of mental health disciplines in the service of restrictive and repressive ideologies – all these have forced us to become more aware of the importance of considering values in our work.

Despite the increasing awareness of the need to recognize, articulate, and transmit values in counselling, there is an oddly persistent notion that our work is value-free. The phrase 'non-judgmental attitude' tends to be interpreted as 'value-free attitude'. During our training we have all learned and often adopted rules such as, 'Avoid moralistic judgments'. In the course of our training all of us, I suppose, have blushed (if we were sensitive) or blanched (if we were devoted) when a supervisor has intoned, as if an anathema: 'You have no right to impose your values on your patient'.

It would not, I think, be amiss for us to pause to examine this statement, so splendidly rhetorical and so readily passed on as from hand to hand, generation to generation. Curiously enough the statement is itself an ethical dictum, with a judgment involved: 'It is *wrong* for the mental health worker to impose his values . . . ' It is also imperative, with a demand involved: 'The mental health worker *must not* impose, etc.' Explicit sanctions may be lacking, but an implied sanction is clear: 'If you say that sort of thing I will be cross with you'. (And, heaven knows, we are frightened to death of making our supervisors cross. Don't you remember the fantasy you had of their career-breaking power over you?)

How curious. The basic aphorism of apparently value-free mental health work is fully moral with content, demand, judgment, and implicit punishment.

But there is no real reason to despair! A cursory examination of the statement's logic shows it to be meaningless. It says, in effect, 'It is a valuable activity not to impose values'. Evidently the sheer non-imposition of values is in some way an imposition of values.

In mental health work we cannot escape from values. Four features call for our consideration today: the impact of values upon our work; the nature of

S. H. Fine, R. Krell, and Tsung-yi Lin (Eds.), 'Today's Priorities in Mental Health' 145–154.

those values; the means by which we, consciously or thoughtlessly, transmit values; and their sources.

II. THE IMPACT OF VALUES ON PRACTISE

London (1967) says aptly:

> Students of mental health find that it is difficult even to *define* such terms as 'health', 'illness', and 'normality', without some reference to morals; and worse still, they cannot discuss the proper treatment of what they have defined without recognizing and involving their own moral commitments.

1. *Values in Assessment and Diagnosis*

By our values we discern abnormalities in mental state. We claim too much for our clinical expertise if we attribute to ourselves detached, objective, 'scientific' powers of observation that no more rely upon values than 18th century Deists relied on God. Szasz (1960) comments, "The notion of mental symptom is . . . inextricably tied to the *social* (including *ethical*) *content* in which it is made in much the same way as the notion of bodily symptom is tied to an *anatomical* and *genetical context*."

What constitutes a delusion? A *false* belief, we say. But 'false' by what criteria? Or: a patient cannot pursue long term goals, form lasting relationships, profit from his experiences, or defer pleasure. But why should he do any of those things? Values that esteem goal-setting, intimacy, conscience, and abstemiousness are clearly to the fore in our assessment of character traits.

Or think for a moment of the immense moral significance of phrases like 'reality testing' or 'out of contact with reality'. We recall that Jesus' family and friends said in alarm, 'He is mad'. His enemies were less flattering: 'He has a devil'. Yet the Christian Church, with a curious perversity in the light of such on-the-spot assessments, has adored Him with one voice as 'My Lord and my God'. One group thought He was out of contact with reality; another has proclaimed for twenty centuries that in Him we confront an Ultimate Reality.

I am not for a moment suggesting that we stop our work of assessment: the pain of humanity will not allow us that sort of high-minded philosophical luxury: but I am suggesting that we acknowledge our assessing and diagnosing as value-determined behaviour. In the mere making of a diagnosis we rely on and we pass on values.

2. *Values and Treatment*

Various workers have noted that value systems are inherent in all psychotherapy. Rollo May (1953) says, "The lack of value judgment which the older therapy opted for is based on a definite philosophical system – that of a fairly complete relativism." And London (1967), ". . . it is apparent that so-called moral neutrality in the psychotherapist is as much a moral position as any more blatant one. It is, from the therapist's side, a libertarian position . . ." Pattison (1968) goes further: "Rather than being amoral, psychotherapy has always been a moral enterprise, and morality has been the central issue of psychotherapy. The psychotherapist *does* and *must* transmit his morality to the patient and influences the morality of his patient." Hartmann (1959) notes moral issues arising in the course of analysis:

> Many patients go through a phase in analysis in which the technical rules that govern the psychoanalytic process are considered, by the patient, as a kind of moral code. . . . This we understand as a transference phenomenon. . . . The analyst's insistence that the patient adhere to certain rules of a technical nature may become a moral demand for the patient . . . The avoidance of what we consider moral value judgments . . . is taken as a model by the patient who tries, thus, to avoid moral value judgment in his own dealing with other people. All this we theoretically expect to come to an end with the termination of a successful analysis. But with some patients it does not.

In psychotherapy, the technical medium is the moral message. It should not surprise us that Watson says bluntly, "An amoral psychotherapy is a contradiction in terms" (Watson 1958).

III. VALUES SUBSERVING COUNSELLING

We have exposed at some length the untenability of the statement, 'The mental health worker does not have the right to impose his values'. How did we come by such a piece of chop-logic? Presumably because it is a rhetorical, if illogical, vehicle of handing on values we have found necessary in effective maintenance of mental health. These values are founded on, and derived from, a belief in the dignity and worth of man, a dignity to be seen in every human individual whom we meet. Much of the time we assume this dignity – for it is often much more an object of faith than of sight. Sometimes, I regret, we forget it; occasionally, God forgive us, we violate it. But in our best moments, sometimes moments of illumination, we know the uniqueness in the universe of this woman, this man who "in all the unrepeatable reality of what he is and what he does, of his intellect and will, of his conscience and heart" (Pope John Paul II 1979) is to be valued for his or her sheer humanity.

We believe that if we are to provide good care we must accept and respect the patient, including his own values, whatever their divergence from our own. We 'willingly suspend disbelief' so that we can, as completely as possible, enter into the world of the patient.

Linked with acceptance are those remarkably value-laden attitudes Carl Rogers has taught us: unconditional positive regard and empathy. Empathy is nowhere better stated than in the second of the great Commandments, "Thou shalt love thy neighbour as thyself." It is always encouraging to a theologian that Rogers offers his definition of 'unconditional positive regard' in theological terms:

> It means a kind of love for the client as he is, providing we understand the word love as equivalent to the theologian's term "agape," and not in its usual romantic and possessive meanings. What I am describing is a feeling which is not paternalistic, nor sentimental, nor superficially social and agreeable. It respects the other person as a separate individual, and does not possess him. (Rogers 1970)

Pope John Paul II is more straightforward in his comments:

> Man cannot live without love. He remains a being that incomprehensible for himself, his life is senseless, if love is not revealed to him, if he does not encounter love, if he does not experience it and make it his own, if he does not participate intimately in it. (Pope John Paul II 1979)

Closely connected with our belief in the dignity of man is our further belief that we must allow another the same right we claim for ourselves, to possess a coherent, motivating, uncoerced value system. We are heirs to a well-developed belief in freedom of conscience. In the English-speaking world it was a somewhat intemperately zealous Baptist who first spoke for full liberty of conscience:

> Our lord the king is but an earthly king, and he hath no authority as a king but in earthly causes, and if the king's people be obedient and true subjects, obeying all human laws made by the king, our lord and king can require no more: for men's religion to God is betwixt God and themselves; the king shall not answer for it, neither may the king be judge between God and man. Let them be heretics, Turks, Jews, or whatsoever, it appertains not to the earthly power to punish them in the least measure. (Helwys 1961)

I need not remind you how reluctantly western civilization accepted this value, how suspicious Christianity was in both its ancient and its reformed wings. The suffering of humble Christians of nonconformist traditions, and of the Jews, won this value for us; the Age of Reason gave it powerful defense; it was accepted belatedly but nobly by the Second Vatican Council. It is cruelly fragile.

We hold, further, that men and women must have a freedom of choice. Redlich (1976) argues persuasively that the fundamental ethical requirement of psychiatry is fully informed consent. Although the major theoretical systems of counselling theory have in them a logical denial of freedom of choice (need I remind you how determinist most 20th century 'scientific' personality theories are?) we have learned that therapy based on those theories is really only effective if the person is well motivated – i.e. has a sense of freedom in choosing to enter and to remain in therapy. In contrast, encumbering mental health work with political ideology is abhorrent to most mental health workers for its denial of human freedom.

The idea that we are free entails a correlative value: that we are responsible. Few values have had more difficulty, or more resilience, in modern psychological theory and technique than human responsibility. The ideas of psychic determinism and unconscious motivation offered a radical challenge to ethics based on human conscious rationality. It is to the credit of Mowrer, of Glasser, of Frankl, and of Dabrowski that they have recognized human responsibility as a major force in modifying behaviour. They see the need to foster responsibility in our treatment modalities, and the necessity of taking freedom and responsibility fully into account in our personality theories.

Hope is another value that generously motivates us in our care of the mentally ill. We engage in our time-consuming, frustrating, slow, arduous work because we believe that men and women can change, not as goal-directed automata, but as persons open to the future when their impediments are removed. Hence many of our approaches are based upon the difficulties of the past, not for archaeological interest, but in order to exorcise that past, to secure remission of it, to win the promise of the heritage of human dignity in a fuller way. C. S. Lewis was no patron of the mental health movement, but he had a deep understanding of the human person and of the human predicament and of human possibilities:

> There are no *ordinary* people. You have never talked to a mere mortal. Nations, cultures, arts, civilisations – these are mortal, and their life is to ours as the life of a gnat. But it is immortals whom we joke with, work with, marry, snub, and exploit – immortal horrors or everlasting splendours. . . . Next to the Blessed Sacrament itself, your neighbour is the holiest object presented to your senses. (Lewis 1965)

That view of man is not only fraught with immense dignity, but also is invested with great hope.

These and other values we cherish; by them we live and care for the emotionally and mentally distressed. And these values are not only deeply human, but profoundly religious.

IV. THE COUNSELLOR AS TRANSMITTER OF VALUES

From the process of value and character formation the mental health worker is mercifully not immune. Indeed we normally have a highly developed and internalized value system. By this internalized value system we hold that what is true (and by that we always mean more than 'descriptively accurate') is good, and therefore binding upon ourselves. The same value system informs us that the false is evil, and to be avoided. We hold that to be true is worthy of ourselves as humans, and so we speak of intellectual integrity, professional ethics, and moral courage as essential professional traits. The true and the false: good and evil: what is befitting the human and what betrays humanity – these are both ethical and religious questions.

A value system has become incorporated as part of our identity. Our human existence is so bound up with values that when we have been persuaded of them, and internalized them, we live by them, we practise our professions by them, we persuade others of them.

Precisely because we are persuaders, transmitters of values, those values must be open to our scrutiny. The process of internalizing values unfortunately renders their scrutiny at once more difficult and more urgent. Since our decisions and actions have values at their heart, neither we nor our clients should expect to escape their impact. All of us who counsel have an obligation to our clientele to examine and to articulate our value systems.

We have a large repertoire of means by which we hand our values on. We are transmitters of values as models. For far too long we have thought we could split our professional values and our personal values. But that splitting is quickly spotted by those who follow us as models. And if the discrepancies are great we lose credibility as mental health workers. As an example – it is possible to have a bad or broken marriage and to be a good marriage therapist. But it is much harder for such a therapist to avoid pathological over-identifications. And, as a pastor, I know that our clientele have grave doubts whether someone who cannot keep his own marriage together can effectively help those whose marriages are falling apart. The laity may not be right technically: they are surely right morally: they are responding to moral issues in the situation: and the central issue is the discrepancy between what happens in the office and at home. If our personal living is narcissistic, we should not be surprised to discover that our patients are behaving in progressively more narcissistic ways.

We pass values along as teachers. We hand on our values not only by our approach to the patient, but also by our treatment of the student. Are we faithful to the humanity of our students? Do we treat them with dignity, with a sense of their worth, as free? Do we hope in them and for them? Do we accept and cherish them? Conveying warmth to patients and abrasiveness or indifference to students; behaving as if patients are of great personal worth but students a beastly nuisance – these discrepancies are too great for students to bear. They learn cynicism quickly. And if we pollute our values with cynicism we become agents of nihilism, not of health.

We transmit values by the theories we construct. Like other intellectual purists I cringe at 'pop-psychology'. But often the various popular forms of the psychologies articulate values more clearly – if more crudely – than the parent theory. So we see narcissism laid bare in much of the self-actualizing popular literature; and hedonism, in pop-analytic theories; and authoritarianism in the popular confrontational schools.

V. RELIGION, THE MENTAL HEALTH WORKER, AND THE TRANSMISSION OF VALUES

I have been suggesting by inference, almost since the beginning of this paper, that we cannot talk about values without beginning to use religious language. None of the values we have mentioned originated with modern mental health movements; none of them emerged in the modern era. The great religions have given richer account of values than we can. Even when we try to construct secular theories and therapies, religious language is upon us (as, for example, in Frankl's work with its many disclaimers to being religious).

Whence these deep values that counsellors profess to hold, or ought to? From Greece. From Palestine. From Italy. The Ionian religio-philosophical constructs;

the Judaeo-Christian tradition; the Renaissance synthesis have each contributed immeasurably to both the content and the structure of our values.

In the west, the healing arts have their philosophical origins in the work of Hippocrates whose work redounded with religion and values, with careful observation and compassionate concern for the welfare of the patient, and with concern for the recovery of an ecological balance between 'nature' and the afflicted. In the west the Greek viewpoint, through its Platonic and Aristotelian refinements, was slowly assimilated to the Judaeo-Christian tradition. The Judaeo-Christian revelational tradition rests upon the fundamental moral statement: "Thou shalt love the Lord thy God with all thy heart, and with all thy soul, and with all thy strength, and with all thy mind; and thy neighbour as thyself." (St. Luke 11 : 27) In the Renaissance the Greek heritage and the Christian ethos were brought to brilliant synthesis after a millenium of debate.

When we analyze the common features of the Greek, the biblical, and the Renaissance views of man we begin to understand the values that inform our work. Each of these sources saw man set apart qualitatively from the environment in which he is integrated. The uniqueness of man – a value much assaulted in these ecological days – qualitatively different from every other object or class of objects in the universe was assumed by the Greek philosophers, accepted by the Renaissance thinkers, and definitely asserted by Judaeo-Christianity with its deep insistence upon man as created in the Image of God – hence profoundly different from every other created object, while in an ecological relationship with all those objects.

A second feature of all these sources of our humane values is their acceptance of man as a being not only unique, but also of immense value. The great Greek tradition deified man in its Pantheon; the Renaissance celebrated man in its arts; and the Judaeo-Christian tradition says in one of its greatest poems:

> When I look at thy heavens, the work of thy fingers,
> the moon and the stars which thou hast established;
> what is man that thou art mindful of him,
> and the son of man that thou dost care for him?
> Yet thou hast made him little less than God,
> and dost crown him with glory and honour. (Psalm 8 : 3–5)

The Christian doctrine of salvation, which is explicitly a doctrine of wholeness, celebrates the grandeur of man – "God so loved the world that He gave His only begotten Son . . ." (St. John 3 : 16) and raises it to new heights in the Incarnation.

Third, all recognize the deep ambivalence of man. This divine dust is sometimes very dusty indeed. Lofty Zeus is a very big, very bad daddy! Man is capable of heaven or hell, as Dante, greatest poet of the west, and supreme poet of the Renaissance so chillingly outlined. Man is a sinner, the biblical tradition says bluntly. Almost no statement so plainly defines the human dilemma as St. Paul's, "All have sinned and come short of the glory of God." (Romans 3 : 23) No existentialist has uttered the pain of this dilemma so movingly as the same Apostle, "For I do not do the good I want, but the evil I do not want is what I do." (Romans 7 : 19)

Fifth, these great traditions have recognized that change is possible, but requires the initiative of another to effect redemption. Very different ideas of redemption have been suggested. Plato argues for an elitist society as redeemer in *The Republic*. The Renaissance argues for learning the scholarship – redemption by the new priesthood of the University. The Judaeo-Christian tradition asserts that God Himself is alone capable of intervening successfully in the tragedy of man, in miracles of grace, by participating completely in our anguish; by being overcome by it, and yet without Himself being smirched by our sin. The Christian dogma of the Incarnation is an inexhaustible fountain of wholeness.

Ultimately, these human values are sustained in all the western traditions by a Blessed Vision. The Platonic vision aspires to Universal Forms; the Aristotelian, to the unmoved Mover; in Dame Juliana of Norwich, Renaissance worldliness gives way to a meek perception of our Courteous Lord; in St. John of the Cross all sense yields to God; in Dante of Florence, grace leads to an ultimate insight that sustains the richest of the values:

> O grace abounding, whereby I presumed
> So deep the eternal light to search and sound
> That my whole vision was therein consumed!
>
> In that abyss I saw how love held bound
> Into one volume all the leaves whose flight
> Is scattered through the universe around. (Dante)

We cannot escape it: mental health work is derived from religion; it is rooted in values bequeathed by religion. With such a heritage the challenge to us is to be faithful to those values that make men whole, and to drink at their sources. We can no longer treat religion as of antiquarian interest. The resurgence of religion in era after era when it has seemed to be superceded by something better – Reason, Humanism, the Classless Society, Self-Actualization, Technique – should make us wary of any quick dismissal of religion as a socially conditioned illusion, or as a transient social phenomenon to be studied as an anthropological curiosity. Religion has given us our values. Can we afford to ignore or despise it? As St. Peter said to Jesus, "To whom shall we go? You have the words of eternal life."

Societies robbed of religion reveal only too quickly their hunger not only for the experience of grace, but for the humanization of the values that religion in its finest hours has articulated, and in its dogmas guaranteed, and in its institutions transmitted.

A religion that came from the East and has shaped the West gives us a splendid set of values:

> He has showed you, O man, what is good;
> and what does the LORD require of you
> but to do justice, and to love kindness,
> and to walk humbly with your God? (Micah 6 : 8)

The supreme exemplar of these values, Jesus Christ, Son of God and Saviour, showed how these became the agenda of wholeness, and that in their activation God reigns:

> And he answered them, 'Go and tell John
> what you have seen and heard: the blind
> receive their sight, the lame walk, lepers
> are cleansed, and the deaf hear, the dead
> are raised up, the poor have good news
> preached to them. And blessed is he who
> takes no offence at me.' (St. Luke 7 : 22, 23)

Clinical Associate Professor of Psychiatry,
Principal of Carey Hall,
University of British Columbia,
Vancouver, B.C., Canada

REFERENCES

Dante Alighieri
The Comedy: Cantica III, Paradise, (Trans. D. L. Sayers and B. Reynolds), Canto XXXIII.

Hartmann, H.
1959 Psychoanalysis and Moral Values, New York: International Universities Press, Inc.

Helwys, T.
1961 A Short Declaration of the Mystery of Iniquity. London 1612 quoted in A. C. Undersood, A History of the English Baptists. p. 47, London: Carey Kingsgate Press.

Lewis, C. S.
1965 The Weight of Glory, in Screwtape Proposes a Toast, and other pieces, p. 109, London: Fontana Books.

London, P.
1967 The morals of psychotherapy, in Mowrer, O. H. (ed.), Morality and Mental Health, Chicago: Rand McNally.

May, R.
1953 Historical and philosophical presuppositions for understanding therapy, in Mowrer, O. H. (ed.), Psychotherapy, Theory and Research, New York: Ronald Press.

Pattison, E. M.
1968 Ego morality: an emerging psychotherapeutic concept. Psychoanal. Rev. 55: 187–222.

Pope John Paul II
1979 Redemptor Hominis. March 15.

Rogers, C. R.
1970 The Interpersonal Relationship: the core of guidance, in Robert T. Golembiewski and Arthur Blumberg (ed.), Sensitivity Training and the Laboratory Approach: readings about concepts and applications, pp. 157–166. Itasca, Ill.: F. E. Peacock Publishers.

Redlich, F. & Mollica, R. V.
1976 Overview: Ethical issues in contemporary psychiatry. Am. J. Psychiatry 133: 125–136.

Szasz, T.
1960 The myth of mental illness. Amer. Psychol. 15:113–118.

Watson, G.
1958 Moral issues in Psychotherapy. Amer. Psychol. 13:574–576.

SECTION SIX

WORKSHOP REPORTS

INTRODUCTION

This section reflects the essence of the Congress. Workshops provide the opportunity for a more intimate exchange of information between Congress participants. It may be of interest to note the format.

For three consecutive days, registrants commit themselves to a workshop of two hours' duration daily. This format provides continuity and participants are able to pursue their ideas into greater depth and details as compared to causal attendance of a variety of workshops.

The size varies from approximately five to twenty-five participants, depending on interest. Each workshop section has a co-ordinator and rapporteur and the following summaries describe their overview of the workshop for which they assumed responsibility.

S. H. Fine, R. Krell, and Tsung-yi Lin (Eds.), 'Today's Priorities in Mental Health' 157.

NANCY DONALDSON, R.N., M.S.N. (U.S.A.) and
OLGA MARATOS, Ph.D. (Greece)

BONDING, ATTACHMENT, AND EARLY INFANT DEVELOPMENT

Parent-infant bonding and attachment is one of the most vital of human relationships. In examining this topic, participants in this workshop considered infant and child development from a variety of cultural and theoretical perspectives. Also explored were the roles of institutions and communities in nurturing optimal beginning relationships between parents and their newborn.

As the family is a dynamic, evolving, and open system, factors influencing bonding and attachment are complex. They include elements which are internal and external to the maternal-infant dyad. There is, for example, a close connection between socio-economic development and family life. Countries suffering from adverse socio-economic conditions are likely to exhibit high rates of perinatal mortality, morbidity, and malnutrition. In such circumstances, promotion of breast-feeding is seen as essential, not only to enhance bonding but also to reduce morbidity and mortality in early infancy.

In cultures with multi-generational living patterns, the quality of attachment in an extended family setting seems not to differ significantly from the quality of attachment found in countries with a nuclear family pattern. The crucial factor, however, may be the consistency of primary attachment figures. Anxiety and overdependence are found in children at the age of puberty when there were experiences of loss, or of multiple mothering.

In observing the process of maternal-infant attachment across cultures, there is evidence to suggest that with attachment, there is dependence. The Japanese term 'Amae' is representative of this concept.

A review of pediatric practice in the developed countries of the world shows that strict schedules in infant care may severely hamper bonding. The age of the mother, at the time of her child's birth, may be another important risk factor. Very young motherhood is often accompanied by an array of adverse psycho-social conditions which affect maternal-infant interaction in early life. These effects are subsequently observed in the development of school-aged children.

Separation from the mother, when a child begins nursery school or kindergarten, can be very upsetting. Studies show that some responses of children are age specific, while other responses seem to be influenced by a child's previous experience of bonding. Multiple mothering may affect the way children react to this separation.

A study of working mothers in the country of Kuwait concluded that the

S. H. Fine, R. Krell, and Tsung-yi Lin (Eds.), 'Today's Priorities in Mental Health' 159–161.

mother's work was not a high risk factor in the development of the children. The impact of a mother's working status, however, may need to be considered within the context of cultural characteristics. There is emerging data to indicate that the infant child is a capable and a very active human being, not only responding to, but also stimulating, the bonding process. Effects of early separation from the mother (postpartum) have behavioral sequelae that are apparent very early in the child's life.

When newborn infants and their mothers experience immediate postpartum separation, sensitive on-going intervention must facilitate the mother's critical bond to her child. Changing the institutional organization, and heightening professional awareness are needed to minimize traumatic effects of early maternal-infant separation. Sensitization of all perinatal personnel should be a continuing process.

Research is needed to determine more clearly how the quality of early parent-child relationships affects later mental development. The effects of psychopathological behavior on the attachment process and parent-child relationships is another area which needs further study. Evidence would suggest, for example, that possessive and narcissistic elements in parental behaviour can compromise the mental health of children.

When therapeutic intervention is necessary for emotionally disturbed infants, it should be recognized that the mother is probably the best therapeutic agent to help her child. At this early stage of development, the therapist should try to optimize self-regulatory mechanisms in the infant.

From a parental point of view, there is the universal need of expectant parents for education and support throughout the child-bearing years. Of great importance are the roles of formal and informal, and professional and non-professional, support systems. The National Childbirth Trust in the United Kingdom offers a useful operational model of these concepts.

The role of the Health Visitor in the United Kingdom is one example of a community service for promoting healthy parent-child relationships. The Health Visitor must be sufficiently trained and sensitized to concepts of bonding and attachment. The contribution of the Health Visitor in providing postpartum follow-up, support, and health education would be vital not only for prevention or early detection of risk factors but also for the continuing monitoring and promoting of maternal-infant bonding. There is need to assign a more active role to people within the community, professional and non-professional, to help families. A useful development would be parent-to-parent support groups, which would serve to balance against the over-professionalization of support given to families.

In conclusion, the majority of participants in this workshop endorsed two recommendations:

(1) Active support for breast-feeding of infants for at least the first six months of life; and

(2) Continuing efforts to promote maximum maternal-infant contact immediately postpartum through rooming-in, or through other similar practices.

RESOURCE PERSONS

Dr. Y. O. Alanen (Finland)
Dr. Sonya Coulin (Germany)
Madame Jacqueline Devooght (Belgium)
Dr. Takeo Doi (Japan)
Dr. Mohamed A. Ghali (Egypt)
Miss Shirley Goodwin (UK)
Dr. Anja Riitta Lahikainen (Finland)
Dr. Lotte Schenk-Danzinger (Austria)
Dr. Benjamin Spock (USA)
Dr. Nebiat Tafari (Ethiopa)
Dr. Sritham Thanaphum (Thailand)
Ms. Penny Wade (UK)

BARBARA KEELEY (UK) and DAVID S. FREEMAN, D. S.W. (Canada)

ALTERNATIVES TO THE NUCLEAR FAMILY: THE ROLE OF THE EXTENDED FAMILY AND THE COMMUNITY IN CHILD REARING

The workshop, Alternatives to the Nuclear Family: The Role of the Extended Family and the Community in Child Rearing concentrated on the following areas:

1. The value of the extended family.
2. The creation of substitute families as an extension of family therapy.
3. Nuclear and extended family's supports in the after care of schizophrenic and/or mentally ill patients.
4. Families in a transitional society.
5. The growth of extensions of the nuclear family through the use of self-help preschool play groups.

The first day of the workshop, the papers focused on demonstrating the key role played by the nuclear family in matters of mental health. The role of the extended family was recognized as more significant than might appear at first sight. It was recognized that in the urbanized societies of developing countries, it asserted a strong influence on its members. Sometimes it performed a malevolent role, bequeathing problems that were worked out in the relationships of later generations or generating conflicts in societies where customs were changing rapidly. Other times the influence was benevolent, with residue or replicated extended families giving support to families with young children, particularly in times of crisis and reinforcing an awareness of the family's self image. In addition, reconstitutions of both nuclear and extended families, based on social rather than blood relationships, were proving effective both therapeutically and in day-to-day living.

The second day of the workshop dealt with the involvement of volunteers in the life of the nuclear and extended family. Two papers pointed out that the breakdown of the extended family brought about by social mobility and urbanization has created a dependency on professional services. In the Philippines, Australia, Britain and the U.S.A., this dependence on professionals is being reduced by an increasing use of volunteers. Sometimes the use of volunteers depended on a simple matching of supply and need, such as the 'adopt a granny' program in the United States in which elderly people were linked with institutionalized mentally retarded children on a one-to-one basis. Both the children and the elderly were enriched by the developing relationships. In other cases,

S. H. Fine, R. Krell, and Tsung-yi Lin (Eds.), 'Today's Priorities in Mental Health' 163–165.

volunteers were prepared for their work by courses, e.g. by year-long, one day a week courses, as in Western Australia. The workshop participants pointed out that the family-replacing potential of the volunteer in self-helping sectors would not be fully realized until three developments occurred:

1. Recognition and acceptance by professionals of the value of self-help in voluntary groups and consequent contribution to the development of support systems for them.
2. Training of professionals for work with volunteers and self-help groups with the emphasis on developing self-reliance rather than dependency upon professionals.
3. Organization of volunteers to increase their accessibility to professionals.

The last day of the workshop focussed on the creation of substitute families as a natural support to families. Two papers stimulated discussion on the creation of substitute families. The first dealt with the creation of a substitute nuclear family for therapeutic purposes in America, the other with the emergence of a substitute extended family as a result of community cooperation in the play groups of Britain.

Substitute therapeutic families opened up new opportunities for family members whose insights into their own problems were inhibited by their real family's situation and relationships. Interest was shown in a program which drew together an interdisciplinary resource group (the therapeutic team) which adopted the roles of nuclear family members. Success seemed to rest upon selecting team members who could empathize with each other; a readiness to learn was as important as relevant experience. Once the therapeutic team was formed, the relationships within the team were welded by constant sharing of thoughts and insights so that teamwork grew from an orchestration of resources. Constant sharing of observations and thought processes between team members of different disciplines diminished reliance on any single member of the group.

Concentration on the child rather than the family of origin was questioned by workshop participants. However, the presenter emphasized that the aim was the reinstitution of true family relationships. One of the most important points made was that substitute family therapy depended on a general stability of staffing that facilitated the synthesis of insights gained from the different professional approaches.

A paper on play groups in Britain raised questions in the minds of workshop members as to the applicability of play groups to their own communities. Discussion drew out ideas and additional points as follows:

1. It is desirable, from the point of view of the mothers, to have very local play groups so that cost of transportation is minimal.
2. Difficulties are created by the situation in which older children are

needed to care for babies while mothers work in the field. In such a situation, it might prove beneficial to have foster play groups in which the older children were learning themselves while playing with the younger ones.

3. The idea of using cooperative play groups to recreate in unstable areas of cities the relationships that exist in stable communities was thoughtfully considered by several members of the workshop.

SUMMARY

There was a general appreciation of the impact of both nuclear and extended families upon the mental health and well-being of individuals. With its less intense relationships, the extended family could be a support to the nuclear family but may also prove to be a threat. If its effect were to replace the nuclear family or create conflict between family members, it could become a menace.

Where mobility in society dispersed extended families, substitute family relationships could be encouraged. These less intense relationships can perform some of the roles of the extended family and also become a resource to the extended family in its efforts to deal with emotional, physical, and social turmoil.

RESOURCE PERSONS

Dr. S. H. Fogel (USA)
M. F. El-Islam (Qatar)
G. Koptagel-Iial (Turkey)
J. Neubauser (Austria)
S. Dihoff (USA)
L. Gillis (South Africa)
R. Cropper (New Zealand)
T. Castelo (Philippines)

EVA BENE, Ph.D. (Canada)

DIVORCE, SEPARATION, AND CUSTODY

Participants at this workshop came from many countries, thus providing an opportunity to examine divorce laws in various parts of the world. Two formal papers were given on the social and psychological stresses experienced by persons undergoing divorce and separation, and these provided a basis for the participants to consider the roles which may be played by mental health workers.

Participants obtained the following information about divorce laws in different parts of the world:

AUSTRIA

More than ten thousand marriages are dissolved each year in Austria, and twelve thousand to fourteen thousand children are affected. A new divorce law, enacted on January 1, 1979, makes it possible for a marriage to be dissolved even against the wishes of one of the marital partners, if they have lived separately for six years. There is little provision for marital counselling apart from help which is available through the Church. Many people seek help from medical practitioners as if they were ill. Some, who are desperate, become alcoholics, and some even commit suicide. If separated parents cannot agree on the fate of their children, a decision is then left to a judge. More often than not, children are given to their mothers.

GERMANY

Germany enacted a new divorce law in 1977. A divorce comes into effect only after custody of children and financial arrangements have been decided. Recently, more attention is being given to the welfare of children involved in divorce cases. A judge may discuss their fate with them regardless of the age of the children, but this is a mandatory procedure if a child is fourteen or over.

SWEDEN

In Sweden, couples with children who contemplate divorce must wait six months, this being a period set aside for thinking things over. If, after the six months, the parents still wish a divorce but cannot decide who should have the children, they can secure psychiatric help. If this still does not result in a decision, then it becomes a matter for the court. A recent law, passed in 1978, provides for the possibility of joint custody of children. This might mean, for example, that a

S. H. Fine, R. Krell, and Tsung-yi Lin (Eds.), 'Today's Priorities in Mental Health' 167–170.

child spends one week with the father and the next with the mother. Such an arrangement can only function, however, if the parents remain good friends. A 'children's telephone' is a special type of service in Sweden. A child who is in trouble can phone for help or for advice and, if necessary, the child will be seen by a social worker. In seeking help, the child can remain anonymous. Last year, over 50 percent of the children who used the 'children's telephone' service did so because their parents were involved in divorce.

LEBANON

In Lebanon, there are very few divorces, but when one occurs, it is handled by the religious community to which the couple belongs. Roman Catholics and Mennonites cannot divorce. There are many marriages in this country which no longer function well; they are referred to as 'empty-shell marriages'. In these situations, there is no communication between the partners, either because they hate one another or because they are totally indifferent. The reason these marriages do not become formally dissolved is because of a high respect for the family as an institution, and a respect for one's religion.

NETHERLANDS

Divorce rates in this country have nearly doubled over the past ten years. In approximately one-half of the cases, there are difficulties involving children and/or financial matters. Decisions about the children are made usually about six months after the divorce. If necessary, the services of a social worker or psychiatrist are used. Children who are aged fourteen or over must be heard by the court; and recently, a bill has been introduced to Parliament to lower this age to twelve. In most cases, children show a preference for the parent with whom they wish to live. However, there often are difficulties with access as the parents may not be willing to cooperate with each other. They might go for family therapy if they can afford it. There are organizations to help those who cannot afford a psychiatrist but there are not enough. With couples who were never legally married, a separation usually finds the mother keeping the children while the father keeps the house; and both are frequently unhappy with such arrangements. There are now various pressure groups trying to improve the family laws of this country.

CANADA (PROVINCE OF BRITISH COLUMBIA)

The Family and Juvenile Courts in this province were combined in 1973. Legal services, counselling, and other social help became more readily available with this change, thus making it possible to establish an atmosphere of trust; clients welcomed the opportunity to be able to explore their conflicts and to consider alternatives to divorce. In the case of broken marriages, the end result is often a legal separation agreement encompassing maintenance, custody of children and access, and the occupation of the home. The courtroom is available to those clients who are unable or unwilling to agree on the issues. If a case does come to court, a new counsellor is appointed as the previous one is bound by confidentiality regarding his discussions with the client. The courts also have resident family advocates who act on behalf of children on family matters. The family advocate could be involved in the conciliation process before the court hearing as he is working closely with the family counsellor or a social worker. If a case comes to a court hearing, the family advocate functions as a lawyer normally does, calling evidence on behalf of a child or cross-examining witnesses. Some of the Family Courts of the province use the Bene-Anthony Family Relations Test, which can be given to parents and to children who are four years of age or older, and provides indications of the feelings family members have for each other.

STRESS OF DIVORCE AND SEPARATION

The emotional process before, during, and after, a divorce can be very painful. Without sympathetic understanding by others, the person who has been left by a marital partner can become ill and desperate. The idea of self-help groups has recently been introduced for people in divorce situations. In these groups, everyone may have an opportunity to discuss his or her problems. In the presence of others who are in the same difficult situation, problems are often more easily resolved and self-confidence re-established. Mutual encouragement helps people to look towards a new future. The self-help group, with the aid of a trained coordinator, is a powerful method of prevention for people who are at medical risk of becoming, for instance, alcoholic or depressed, or developing psychosomatic diseases.

EFFECTS OF SOCIAL FRAGMENTATION

If we are aiming for good mental health, then we must become aware of the processes of 'inner separation'. These processes, which occur within the individual, usually are not in one's consciousness. Society has been broken up into various fragments of which we are only more or less aware. This fragmentation of society leads to a deformation of our inner life. Our social attitudes also prevent a full awareness of our emotions. In order to achieve real mental health, we must become conscious of all those social processes which are deforming our inner life, even if attempts to achieve such consciousness are very painful.

RESOLUTION

At the conclusion of this workshop, participants unanimously passed the following resolution:

– WHEREAS this workshop is concerned with the effects of an increasing breakdown of marriages;

– WHEREAS the focus of these concerns is the quality of life, particularly with regard to children who are involved; and

– WHEREAS in some countries, potential adoptive parents receive mandatory personal and child-rearing counselling,

Be it resolved that governments be approached through the World Federation for Mental Health to see that all potential parents receive child-rearing counselling, e.g. during the last year of compulsory schooling.

RESOURCE PERSONS

Allison Burnet (Canada)
Eve Bene (Canada)
Rosalee Hardin (Canada)
Marianne Lene (Sweden)
Gretl Pilz (Austrial)
Claus Ritters (West Germany)
H. Wegerif (Netherlands)
Edith Wehle (Austria)

BEN CHUD, M.S.W. (Canada) and RICHARD NANN, D.S.W. (Canada)

MENTAL HEALTH OF CHILDREN OF MIGRANTS AND CULTURAL MINORITIES

Migration of people is not a recent phenomenon; it has occurred throughout human history, is occurring now, and will occur in the future. It follows that members of helping professions will continue to encounter issues and problems arising from human migration.

The topic of this workshop is a continuation of a theme developed at the 1977 World Congress on Mental Health in Vancouver. That previous workshop was concerned primarily with adult members of migrant populations and examined, on the one hand, uprooting problems associated with planned, voluntary movement (e.g., economically-induced immigration) and, on the other, problems associated with unplanned involuntary movement (e.g., politically-induced flight).

In conjunction with the main theme of the 1979 Congress, the current workshop focussed on problems encountered by the children of migrant groups. Based on experiences in six different countries, papers were heard on topics ranging from adaptation of children of immigrant parents, to experiences of families of foreign workers, to problems of visiting students studying in a foreign environment. A number of general conclusions and observations emerged from the workshop discussions and deliberations. These are presented in the remainder of this summary.

PERSONAL PROBLEMS AND SOCIAL ISSUES

The problems of migrant families and children cannot be dealt with in isolation from larger social, political, and economic issues. This point was made very clear when we examined the experiences of immigrant children in the Netherlands, the problems of refugee children in Belgium, and the status of families of migrant workers in Germany. In working with migrant populations, we must be prepared to engage in issues and problems at different levels, whether these are macro (societal), mezzo (local community), or micro (family and individual).

We must be realistic in seeking solutions. Given the complexity of factors which induce movement, it may be more useful to speak of responses to problems associated with uprooting and settlement rather than solutions. This does not mean that we should not aim for solutions in certain instances. For example, we heard an account of psychiatric services in rural Australia which provided help to an immigrant lad who had been sleeping with his mother for several years, and had been a bed-wetter all of this time. It is no small accomplishment to help this boy overcome his problems.

S. H. Fine, R. Krell, and Tsung-yi Lin (Eds.), 'Today's Priorities in Mental Health' 171–173.

THE IMPORTANCE OF LANGUAGE

Language acquisition is a crucial variable in the lives of migrant populations. Immigrants must learn the language of their host society; otherwise they remain socially and economically disadvantaged. But language alone does not move immigrants out of the lowest rungs of the economic ladder. Language is not simply a form of communication. In many ways, it is a medium for acquiring values and norms. Moreover, it involves a question of self-image.

Although children of immigrant families may not quickly acquire a high sophistication in the use of a new language, it is often the case that their linguistic skills are far in advance of those of their parents. This often exacerbates the problem of intergenerational conflict among immigrant families.

BELIEF SYSTEMS, VALUES, AND CULTURAL ROOTS

Belief systems, values, and cultural roots run very deep and are very tenacious. This point was emphasized when we heard about the experiences of many Japanese families, living abroad for governmental or for business purposes, whose desire is for their children to maintain their Japanese culture and someday return home to their native land. It is important to keep in mind that the cultural roots of people have evolved over centuries.

In North America as well as in other countries with high rates of immigration, experience has shown that, no matter how the dominant host culture sets out to assimilate immigrants, cultural differences will persist. In acknowledging this phenomenon, the government in Canada has adopted a policy of 'multiculturalism'; and in the United States today, one speaks of 'cultural pluralism'. These policies constitute a sharp shift from a 'melting-pot' approach which, in North America at least, has been more of a theory than actuality.

ADAPTABILITY OF CHILDREN

While it is understandable for mental health workers to be concerned with problems facing immigrant groups, a fact frequently overlooked is that human beings are very adaptable; and children in particular are probably the most adaptable segments of humanity. All children, however, require a healthy environment for growth and maturation. Of particular importance to the immigrant child is his or her experience at school. The school system must provide a congenial atmosphere for the immigrant child, and a crucial factor here is the attitude of teachers. Mental health workers have a vital task in linking immigrant homes to the educational, recreational, and community systems.

Immigrant children are in a special position. They become the transmitters, or go-betweens, of two cultures. If the host country and its educational and socializing institutions can create an atmosphere in which immigrant children are made to feel that they are worthy, and that they and their people are taken into account, then these values are transmitted to the home. If, on the other hand, immigrant children encounter negative experiences, then these, too, are felt in the home. This is why it is so important to deal with the needs of immigrant children at different levels.

Sometimes, we can influence the macro system at the highest level of government. More frequently, breakthroughs can be made at a local or community level. It does not follow, of course, that we will dispense with all problems but, at least, we will have made a contribution by way of preventive activity.

RESOURCE PERSONS

M. C. Fereday (Australia)
Akira Hoshino (Japan)
Patrick Okura (USA)
F. Poustka (Germany)
R. Trevino (Belgium)
Broos Verdonk (The Netherlands)

Prof. Dr PETER BERNER (Austria), CHING-PIAO CHIEN, M.D. (U.S.A)
and JOEL A. MOSKOWITZ, M.D. (U.S.A.)

THE IMPACT ON CHILDREN IN AN OVERMEDICATED SOCIETY

Due to the complexities of the impact on children in an overmedicated society, the main focus was placed on three particular areas of concern: (1) substance abuse, especially alcohol and cigarette smoking; (2) food substances, nutritious and non-nutritious (e.g., enhancers, extenders, coloring); and (3) medicinal agents, prescribed and non-prescribed.

The workshop started with an examination of the definition and magnitude of the problem which is implied by the term 'overmedicated society'. In this regard, a somewhat different perspective was offered by a paper which considered medication problems in the context of an 'undermedicated society'. Specifically, this paper reported on experiences in the rural areas of Mexico where, despite a lack of medical facilities and conventional medicines, the potential for health hazards still existed because of self-medication with herbs and drugs obtained from other than medical resources.

A second paper reviewed the historical antecedents of overmedication patterns in the United States. Reported occurrences of both physical and mental ill effects of many common medicinal agents were noted, as were the impacts of such agents at various stages of child development. The latter include, for example: (a) 'fetal alcohol syndrome' and the small birth weights of infants born to smoking mothers and fathers, (b) hypervitaminosis in infancy, (c) hidden chemicals such as hormones in foods, (d) late carcinogenic effects of estrogen upon offsprings of women given diethylstilbestrol, and (e) substance abuse during adolescence and youth. From a psychiatric and pediatric viewpoint, the overall picture is one of overt and covert health hazards from direct and indirect medication and chemical exposure.

Another paper presented experimental data derived from a crossover, double-blind design, to evaluate the efficacy of Feingold non-food additive for hyperkinetic children. No significant difference was found between the placebo and the experimental group of 16 children. However, one should not overgeneralize from this limited study which used only four food colorings and no flavorings. A future study with a larger sample population and more implicated harmful food substances is desirable.

In the latter part of this workshop, attention was given to the role of governments in regulating the drug market. In this regard, one paper reviewed some historical aspects of governmental involvement in the regulation of drug marketing in the United States. The exposure of children to drugs, and the rights of children

S. H. Fine, R. Krell, and Tsung-yi Lin (Eds.), 'Today's Priorities in Mental Health' 175–176.

were examined. Consumer involvement in legislation and governmental regulation was recommended. Along this line, experiences in Indonesia were presented with particular reference to the new role of expert pharmacologists and toxicologists in screening drugs for governmental approval.

This workshop also viewed a powerful film entitled, *The Feminine Mistake*, which is used as an educational tool by the American Cancer Society. This film emphasizes the dangerous consequences of cigarette smoking on women. Graphic evidence of physiologic harm to the fetus was demonstrated in the case of expectant mothers. Viewers were also alerted to the tragic carcinogenic effects in the adult, as well as the dramatic premature skin wrinkling and blood vessel spasm effects of smoking.

Thus, the workshop addressed its primary concern to the direct impact of substances (habitual, food and medicinal) on the physical and mental health of children. The impact on children in an overmedicated society in terms of personality development, coping mechanism, and their value systems was not dealt with in depth due to the time schedule. However, the workshop acknowledged its importance for future study.

Some intensive discussion took place in the workshop as to possible future solutions. There was general agreement on the following points:

(1) The public needs to be better informed and educated about the hazards of medication and chemical exposure;

(2) Only a responsible, informed, and educated consumer group with knowledgeable expert input can make constructive recommendations to legislators where governmental control is indicated;

(3) There is need for further studies on the psychosocial and cultural aspects of community attitudes towards drugs and chemicals. Based on such data, an approach within the context of each society and culture can then lead to appropriate utilization of effective medications with assurance of maximum physical and mental health.

RESOURCE PERSONS

Dr. Guido Belsasso (Mexico)
Dr. Eduardo Dallal (Mexico)
Dr. Rachel Gittelman (USA)
Dr. Kusumanto Setyonegoro (Indonesia)
Arlene Moskowitz, J.D. (USA)

C. S. IERODIAKONOU, Ph.D. (Greece) and WESLEY SHERA, M.A. (Canada)

EXTERNAL STRESSES ON FAMILY LIFE

This workshop explored the many ways in which various environments such as the community, social institutions, and culture, impact on the life of individuals and families. Through the use of a multi-environmental sectoral analysis, various types and levels of external impacts and their interdependencies were identified.

A suggested model showing the individual and his or her environments is presented at the end of this summary. Within this scheme, the following types and levels of environments are seen as particularly relevant:

(1) The nuclear, or the multi-generation family (tribe);
(2) The participatory environment (once the village or neighborhood);
(3) The community or municipality;
(4) The culture, society, or nation;
(5) The international scene;
(6) The cosmos.

Each of these environments contributes its part to the development of the person; and each, in turn, is potentially influenced by this growing person. The average human being has close family ties, and participates personally in a number of local, or local branches of collectivities such as the village, neighborhood, school, job, or commercial organizations. If he/she is not personally involved with them, he/she sense of a desirable reference group gives the same feeling of belonging as is attained by participating directly. Most residents have some abstract sense of the overall community, especially if they are transformed into voting citizens every few years; and certain citizens may even be active in local affairs. However, only well-developed individuals have any significant appreciation of the more distant environments (national, international, and cosmic); and few play an active role in them. Nevertheless, these three environments have a very powerful impact on the individual's choice of lifestyle, on his opportunity structure, and on his course of developmental growth.

An example was given in a paper examining the impact of public policy on family life in Canada. A recent surge of interest in family policy in this country has led to the parallel development of interest in family impact statements. Assessment of potential effects of policies on families is particularly important today given the current state of the Canadian economy, the current emphasis on fiscal constraints for social programs, and the increasing pressure to identify priorities.

While the growing interest in family policy can be viewed as a step in the right direction, there remains a tendency to restrict attention to policies which have a

S. H. Fine, R. Krell, and Tsung-yi Lin (Eds.), 'Today's Priorities in Mental Health' 177–179.

direct impact on the family. There is need to extend our attention to take into account the pervasive effects that general public policies have on the family (for example, policies reflected in areas like taxation, welfare, resource development, education, etc.). The impact of such policies is often most noticeable when viewed from a multicultural perspective. In Canada, it is often the thirty percent of the population from backgrounds that are neither French nor English who absorb many of the negative consequences of Canadian public policy.

An examination of the Canadian scene from a multicultural perspective can contribute to a global perspective which recognizes the need to explore the impact of international interdependencies. This awareness of the global mosaic will hopefully promote a more serious discussion about the types of national and international policies which truly contribute to human development.

Another paper examined the profound effects that major changes in women's roles have had on family life in the United States. Of particular relevance to this workshop were: (a) increasing participation of women in the labor force; (b) changing patterns of marriage and divorce; and (c) shifting values and practices regarding fertility. Since women have traditionally borne the responsibility for family maintenance and childcare, these changes can be expected to have an important effect on family life, although it is still too early to know precisely the long-term effects.

Changes in women's roles also carry implications for social institutions outside of the family. For example, some immediate impact can be predicted upon community institutions that aid parents in the care, and the socialization, of their children.

A paper examining preventive aspects of children's mental health in Greece offered further illustrations of the importance of sociocultural factors which affect a child's emotional life. Preventive mental health measures for children must include provision for the physical health of the expectant mother, a psychological milieu which offers love and security for the child, and social conditions which help the child to grow and mature as an individual. Drawing on research findings and clinical experiences, this paper reviewed the sociocultural elements in Greek society which help or hinder healthy mental development, taking into account the impact of such factors as: urbanization trends, the attitudes of the Greek family to children, the roles of the Greek mother and grandmother, and the place of the adolescent in the Greek family.

Yet another paper presented to the workshop described some impacts of wartime and natural catastrophies on families in Israel. Use was made of crisis theory to explain such resultant behaviour as: organizational paralysis (especially in the participatory environment), community-wide demoralization, psychosomatic illness, and various frenzied searches for psychosocial security. Attention was devoted to one particular issue – relations between Israeli Arabs and Jews as they face the prospects of living in peace after at least 30 years of fear, misunderstanding, and hostility.

One of the strategies for dealing with the crises and inter-group tensions placed high reliance on principles of community social work practice, as well as on the experience accumulated in Israel by a national voluntary association of Arabs and Jews called 'Partnership'.

The paper also included some speculations as to how families and individuals with initiative might be able to make supportive or remedial impacts on the multiple environments within which they function.

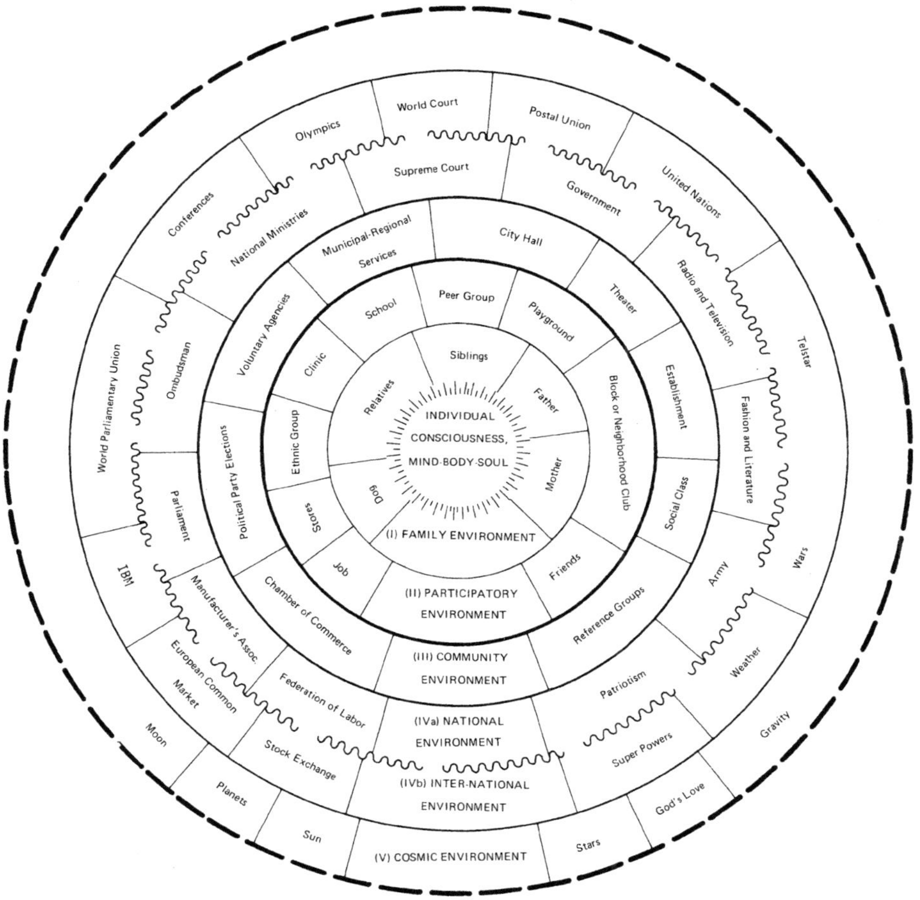

Figure. Individuals and environments: a suggested model.

RESOURCE PERSONS

Jean Kristeller (USA)
Jeanne Marecek (USA)
Benyamin Chetkow-Yanoov (Israel)

BRIAN G. FRASER, J.D. (U.S.A.), Judge JACK E. DOEK (Holland), EDITH LANDO (Canada)

CHILD ABUSE AND NEGLECT

The child abuse and neglect workshop focused on the identification, investigation and intervention (treatment) of suspected child abuse and neglect. The workshop was designed to highlight how different countries accomplish these three steps. The workshop also discussed prediction (a precursor to identification), emphasized the growing problem of sexual abuse, debated various methods of treatment and prevention, and closed with a discussion of a proposal to support an international organization which would work actively on child protection.

The first day of the workshop focused on how America, Netherlands and France deal with child abuse and neglect.

In America the identification and reporting of suspected cases of child abuse is mandated by law. Each state has enacted a mandatory reporting statute. The mandatory reporting statute defines child abuse, identifies various groups of individuals, and mandates that they report suspected cases of child abuse. Reports are made to a state department of social services. That department investigates the suspected case, determines if child abuse is present and provides treatment where necessary. In some cases the department of social services may refer the case to the juvenile court and that court will mandate that treatment be implemented.

In the Netherlands there are no mandatory reporting statutes. Reports of suspected child abuse are made to 'confidential doctors'. There are ten confidential doctors located throughout the country. Upon receipt of a report of suspected child abuse the confidential doctor will conduct an investigation and determine if child abuse is present. The confidential doctor may suggest a certain plan of treatment and provide help in implementing it. If the child abuse is serious the confidential doctor has two additional options. He may suggest that the original reporter file a formal report with the Child Protection Board; or he may file a formal report himself with that Board. The Child Protection Board may conduct its own investigation and may refer the case to the juvenile court for implementation of treatment if he believes that it is necessary.

France, like the Netherlands, has no mandatory reporting statute. In France, unlike the U.S. and the Netherlands, there is no special agency to deal with the problems of child abuse. The two services which deal with abused children are the Department for the Protection of Mothers and Infants and the Child Welfare Services. The Department is responsible for the child to age six. Child health visitors from the Department visit all children, identifying high risk families and abused children. The Child Welfare Services provide aid for families,

S. H. Fine, R. Krell, and Tsung-yi Lin (Eds.), 'Today's Priorities in Mental Health' 181–185.

care for homeless children and protection for the child (i.e. from abuse). France is divided into 90 departments, each having the same services. Treatment can be offered through the Department for Protection of Mothers and Infants, or the Child Welfare Services, or the juvenile court.

Much of the past research dealing with the identification of various forms of child abuse has dealt with evidence of physical trauma inflicted on children. The isolation of certain behavioural and developmental aspects of the abused child, however, coupled with tangible evidence of physical trauma can make the diagnosis and the identification of child abuse a much more accurate process.

It was pointed out that the difficulties of mentally ill parents and their children are closely interwoven. In point of fact, children of mentally ill parents have a much greater likelihood of suffering emotional abuse than the general population. In the past much attention and available resources have been provided to the mentally ill parents. Since the children of these parents are a great risk population, it was suggested that more attention be paid to the children. It was noted that the numbers of children so affected are not so great that resources could not be appropriated to prevent future problems.

The second day of the Child Abuse workshop dealt primarily with sexual abuse. Two papers were presented which dealt with sexual abuse treatment programs and one paper with the criminal law.

It was noted that there is a need to make a clear distinction between sexual abuse, incest, and sexual exploitation. Each has separate diagnostic, assessment and treatment needs. The structure of treatment is of particular importance. Treatment of incest must begin with individual counselling, followed by conjoint counselling and, finally, when all parties are ready, group treatment. Treatment can be successful, but it must be carefully structured.

The second paper agreed that individual treatment is necessary. The primary focus of that treatment, however, should be the child. This program, pioneered in California, has treated over 2000 individuals, primarily in the incest area. Characterized as a 'humanistic' community treatment model, it has three components; a professional component, a volunteer component, a self-help component. This humanistic model has proved so successful that, with federal funding, it will become a national program sometime in 1980.

There was considerable discussion of European Laws and their impact on sexual abuse. A number of suggestions for future action were proposed as the basis of these laws. In particular, it was suggested that a non-punitive approach he taken. Specifically, it was felt that penalty clauses in the criminal law concerning incest could be abrogated (except those cases involving serious physical harm to the child).

Two additional papers were presented on the second day. The first dealt with a study of 36 abused children and their families. A comparison of this group with a control group indicated significant differences. The most pronounced were the mother's perception of the baby, the father's reaction to the birth, the parents' interaction with the child, the amount of supervision and interpersonal actions between both parents and the child. An interesting aspect of this study was the high correlation between premature births and abuse.

The second paper dealt with a study conducted in Finland of 200 children under the age of two, who were seen in an out-clinic service. Particular attention in the study was paid to the child, the type of abuse, and parental isolation as a factor in child abuse.

Most of the discussion on the second day centered around different treatment models for sexual abuse. There was one point of absolute consensus. Treatment, if it is to be effective, must involve the community. It has been shown to be exceptionally effective and very inexpensive.

The third and final day involved discussion of a community program to deal with high risk families, the need to develop a new international ethic, home health visitors, primary prevention, and a proposal to support an international organization for maltreated children.

It was noted that mental health professionals have an opportunity and an obligation to provide child abuse prevention information to professionals working with children. It is now possible to identify high risk families at birth. In point of fact, it was indicated that many maternity staffs do now identify high risk families, but little, if any, follow-up is provided. It was suggested that information about how to identify high risk families be provided to all maternity staffs, and that the proper supportive services be provided following birth. This, it was indicated, would substantially reduce the incidence of child abuse.

The second paper suggested that child abuse was a part of a much larger problem: human violence. Violence, it implied, was learned and taught in the home, the church and the schools. What can be learned can be unlearned. If human violence was substantially reduced, child abuse would be substantially reduced. It is recommended that America, like other countries, should adopt a new national ethic: 'Raise Children Without Hitting'. Reference was made to the new legislation enacted in Sweden against corporal punishment of any kind.

The next paper dealt with the primary prevention of child abuse, that is, ensuring that child abuse never takes place. Primary prevention if it is to be successful, must be based in the community and must be comprehensive. Elements of this comprehensive program should include the areas of: pre-natal programs; perinatal bonding programs; programs in interacting with infants; programs for parents of non-normal infants; home health visitor programs; mutual aid programs, crisis care programs; child care programs; child screening and treatment programs; therapeutic programs for abused children; education for adulthood programs.

The fourth paper dealt with one of the programs referred to in the paper on Prevention – the Home Health Visitor Program in England. Each home health visitor, of which there are approximately 10 000, is a registered nurse and each receives a four month training course before being licensed. All children are visited by the Home Health Visitor 10 days after birth, and then at regular intervals over the next few years. These individuals provide good health care promptly. The participants in the workshop felt that to make this kind of program truly effective community support and additional back-up services would be required.

The final presentation dealt with the creation of a new international organization called DEFENCE FOR CHILDREN. The basic outline of the organization's structure and goals were explained. It was understood that this organization would function on behalf of maltreated children throughout the world. Indicating that other international organizations had formally voiced support for DEFENCE FOR CHILDREN it was proposed that the Child Abuse Workshop prepare a resolution to be brought to the entire WFMH Congress. The proposal was adopted by a voice vote.

RESOLUTION FROM WORKSHOP NO. 7 'CHILD ABUSE AND NEGLECT'

Mrs. Edith Lando, North American Co-ordinator

TO: The Participants at the Congress of the World Federation for Mental Health, held in Salzburg, Austria, July 8–13, 1979

CONSIDERING that child maltreatment, with its implications for mental health, is not purely an intrafamilial phenomenon, but is also perpetrated at all levels of social organization, up to and including governmental agencies;

CONSIDERING that no international organization is currently specifically concerned with setting up and promoting channels at national and international levels for the effective protection and representation of the children concerned;

AWARE that several international humanitarian bodies have expressed the need for an organization of that kind, and that in particular the International Society for the Prevention of Child Abuse and Neglect has stated its intention of collaborating closely with such an initiative;

CONVINCED of the need for permanent and organized international solidarity and action on individual and group cases of child maltreatment that cannot be resolved at the national level;

AWARE of the existence and aims of a newly-established international non-governmental organization in Geneva called Defense for Children, designed to work precisely in this sphere;

BE IT RESOLVED:

– that every effort be made, by concerned individuals and organizations, both national and international, to foster cooperation with Defense for Children and to further its actions and aims;

– The World Federation for Mental Health is requested to recommend to the Executive Board that it study the ways in which it could collaborate with the work of Defense for Children to protect the potential or actual child victims of abuse, neglect and exploitation when international intervention or support is required.

RESOURCE PERSONS

T. Arajarvi (Finland)
Nigel Cantwell (Switzerland)
Henry Ciarretto (USA)
Karen E. Ledger (Canada)
Kenneth N. McRae (Canada)
R. K. Oates (Australia)
Rhoda Oppenheimer (UK)
Pierre Straus (France)
June Thompson (UK)
John E. Valusek (USA)
Alexander Zaphiris (USA)

Dr M. CARBALLO (Switzerland) and GRAYCE M. ROESSLER, R.N., Ph.D. (U.S.A)

FOOD HABITS AND MENTAL HEALTH OF CHILDREN

The Food Habits and Mental Health of Children workshop focussed mainly on the vital role of appropriate and adequate nutrition in the development of physical and mental health of children.

Workshop members emphasized that malnutrition and malnourishment are common throughout the world. It was pointed out that studies demonstrate that good nutrition offers the best protection against disease. Nutritional factors also play an important role in the elevation of verbal intelligence and abstract reasoning of malnourished children.

Mental health in children is closely related to growth changes. At the same time, the influence of physical growth interfaces with mental health. The primary concern of workshop participants was the apparent neglect of mental health workers of the importance of optimal nutrition for children in the development and maintenance of good mental health. The role of environmental factors was discussed. However, the group was most insistent that good nutrition is the basic and primary foundation of good physical and mental health.

During the past few decades, breast-feeding has been continuously declining in most industrialized and many developing societies. Breast-fed children have shown to be better protected against serious intestinal infections, malnutrition, metabolic disturbances, obesity, milk allergies, and many communicable diseases. Also, maternal-infant relationships are demonstrably improved.

Discussions in the workshop centred around the present world-wide trend towards formula and artificial feeding of young infants. Several factors were pointed out concerning the desirability of breast-feeding. They were identified as: the ease of preparation, sterility, availability, inexpensiveness, and others in addition to those previously mentioned. The discussants expressed great concern relative to the world-wide promotion of artificial feedings for infants. Additionally, they advised that environmentalists and health advisors throughout the world examine the impact of the introduction of alien foods into their cultures – food which may have marked and unexpected consequences on cultural values and lifestyles and, most importantly, on survival.

Finally, as health care givers throughout the world are generally perceived as influential in food habits and choices, the group recommended emphatically more intensive and extensive education in nutrition, not only for mental health workers but for all persons providing health education and care.

S. H. Fine, R. Krell, and Tsung-yi Lin (Eds.), 'Today's Priorities in Mental Health' 187–188.

RESOLUTION FROM WORKSHOP NO. 9 'FOOD HABITS AND MENTAL HEALTH OF CHILDREN'

Dr Grayce Roessler, North American Co-ordinator

TO: Executive Committee, WFMH

WHEREAS: During the past few decades, breast-feeding has been continuously declining in most industrialized countries, and many developing societies, and

WHEREAS: Breast-fed children are better protected against serious intestinal infections, malnutrition, metabolic disturbances, obesity, milk allergies, and several communicable diseases, and

WHEREAS: Maternal/infant relationships are shown to be improved through breast-feeding, and

WHEREAS: Breast-feeding remains inexpensive to maintain, and

WHEREAS: Human milk is very different from cows' milk and milk substitutes, and

WHEREAS: Formula and artificial feeding is widely promoted throughout the world and with deleterious effects on infants and their families, and

WHEREAS: Health care givers are perceived as being influential in determining the choice of infant feeding,

THEREFORE BE IT RESOLVED THAT:

- The World Federation for Mental Health actively support breast-feeding of infants for *at least* the first six months of life, and

BE IT FURTHER RESOLVED THAT:

- The World Federation for Mental Health actively support more intensive and extensive education of health care givers relative to the values of breast-feeding, and the World Federation for Mental Health go on record as disapproving commercial interest promotions of artificial formula feeding for young infants throughout the world.

SIGNED: Dr. Horst Schetelig, Germany; Dr. Arthur Kaslow, USA; Dr. Catherine Wenner, Netherlands; Janet Youmans, RN, USA; Barbara Kemp, England; Claude Chemtob, USA; H.I.J. van der Spuy, Canada; and Dr. Grayce Roessler, USA.

RESOURCE PERSONS

Dr. Claude Chemtob (USA)
Dr. D. Evans (South Africa)
Dr. Arthur L. Kaslow (USA)
Dr. H.I.J. van der Spuy (Canada)

SERGE A. DIHOFF, B.A., B.S., PAUL F. FENDT, Ph.D.,
ANNETTE JURGELSKI, M.A.T.

PROBLEMS OF EXCEPTIONAL CHILDREN: THE GIFTED AND THE LIMITED

The special needs of the exceptional child have become a joint concern of the family, the state and society as a whole. To deal effectively with this population of children, a variety of approaches and support systems are needed. This workshop discussed some of the approaches and support systems in current use.

There is evidently widespread interest in providing appropriate programs for children who are handicapped. In West Germany, this concern is manifest by a government action which commissioned a private firm to evaluate and criticize existing programs. The results of the study were distributed at the workshop.

Because society tends to evaluate families on the abilities and successes of their children, a handicapped child may prove a negative (low-rating) factor for the family. Parents and siblings may react with extremes of self-sacrifice, resentment, flight or indifference. Whatever the family response, the handicapped child, inevitably more dependent than the normal child, will be drastically affected. Thus early emotional, pedagogic, social, and financial help to the family may be an essential factor in minimizing the handicap.

By the time the handicapped child reaches adolescence, special assistance is needed to teach the residential and vocational skills necessary for independent living outside the family unit. The Scandinavian countries and, more recently, the United States, have endorsed the Normalization Principle, which asserts that handicapped individuals will attain a higher level of function in a community rather than in an institutional setting. Portugal also has used this approach in some programs for handicapped young people.

Programs based on the Normalization Principle are usually committed to a policy of deinstitutionalization. Handicapped adolescents are encouraged to follow a lifestyle similar to that of their contemporaries in the mainstream of society. They remain residents of the community, follow the usual patterns of work and leisure, and are vocationally trained and employed by local enterprise.

The Caramore Community, a U. S. demonstration project established by the North Carolina Association for the Emotionally Troubled, actively incorporates the Normalization Principle in its rehabilitation program for handicapped young men and women. At Caramore, participants receive training and support which permit them to live and work in the community. Initially, most reside in a supervised group home and work in Caramore-operated enterprises. Ultimately, they progress to independent apartment living and employment by local industry.

S. H. Fine, R. Krell, and Tsung-yi Lin (Eds.), 'Today's Priorities in Mental Health' 189–191.

A professional staff provides instruction, encouragement, and guidance throughout the step-by-step residential and vocational training.

In shaping the behavior of handicapped individuals who are mentally retarded, positive and negative feedback may play as significant a role as in the behavior modification of normal individuals. A study by California State University staff of 32 retarded residents of a hospital in Pomor, California (U.S.A.) showed that individuals with mental age as low as 3.6 years can distinguish between positive and negative reinforcement. The study divided the subject population into four groups and assigned each group the same task to perform. The variable was the type of verbal reinforcement given each group.

Results indicate that greater group cohesiveness – and presumably a more facilitative atmosphere – will result when all feedback given is positive. However, pure negative feedback or positive feedback followed by negative feedback produces greater behavioral impact than pure positive feedback.

Ideally, feedback should be consistent and appropriate to the situation which elicits the response. Although continuous reinforcement schedules may be initially useful to establish the desired behavioral repertoire, a gradual changeover to the more typical intermittent reinforcement is recommended.

If positive interpersonal peer relationships are to be established in a retarded population, the group learning situation such as classroom or workshop may provide an optimal setting. Within this environment, the proper feedback coding may have important implications for making the group attractive and cohesive – two key factors in its effectiveness.

Workshop members apparently concurred in the belief that handicapped children and young people are capable of more than simple functional autonomy. With timely intervention, appropriate instruction and proper reinforcement, these individuals can look forward to a considerable degree of independence and self-determination.

Because presentations dealt exclusively with the problems of the limited child, the discussions tended to emphasize this issue. However, a need for more work on the special needs of gifted children was acknowledged, with the lack of papers cited as possible evidence that this area is being neglected.

RESOURCE PERSONS

V. Benesova (Czechoslovakia)
J. Box van den Broecke (Holland)
S. Dihoff (USA)
I. Emich (Austria)
P. E. Ernstrom (USA)
M. C. Freeberg (USA)
H. Heinemann (Germany)
A. Jacobs (USA)
M. S. Notarius (USA)
G. Orth (Germany)
A. de Smedt (Belgium)
W. Smith Valand (USA)
H. Speierl (Austria)
E. Tutaan (Philippines)
L. Valdez (Philippines)
W. Walcher (Austria)
M. Zapletalek (Czechoslovakia)

REFERENCES

Bandura, A.
1969 Principles of Behaviour Modification. New York: Holt, Rinehart, & Winston.

Dittes, J. E. & Kelley, H. H.
1956 Effects of different conditions of acceptance upon conformity to group norms. Journal of Abnormal Social Psychology 53, 100–107.

Dybwad, Gunnar
1969 "Action Implications in the USA Today" in Changing Patterns in Residential Services for the Mentally Retarded. Edited by R. B. Kagel and W. Wolfensberger. Washington, D. C., President's Committee on Mental Retardation Monograph.

Emery, H. G. and Brewster, K. G. (Eds.)
The New Century Dictionary of the English Language, Vol. 1, New York, P. F. Collier and Son.

Grunewald, Karl
1969 The Mentally Retarded in Sweden. Stockholm: Kugelsbergs, Kohtryckerl AB.

Jacobs, M., Jacobs, A., Feldman, G. & Cavior, N.
1973 "Feedback II: The 'Credibility Gap': Delivery of Positive and Negative Emotional and Behavioral Feedback in Groups" in Journal of Consulting and Clinical Psychology 41, 215–223. a.

Jacobs, M. Jacobs, A., Gatz, M. and Schaible, T.
1973 "Credibility and Desirability of Positive and Negative Structured Feedback in Groups" in Journal of Consulting and Clinical Psychology 40, 244–262. b.

Kelley, H. H. & Shapiro, M. M.
1954 An Experiment on Conformity to Group Norms where Conformity is Detrimental to Group Achievement. American Sociological Review 29, 667–677.

Nirje, Bengt
1969 "The Normalization Principle and Its Human Management Implications" in Changing Patterns in Residential Services for the Mentally Retarded. Edited by R. B. Kagel and W. Wolfensberger. Washington, D. C., President's Committee on Mental Retardation Monograph.

Rose, S. D.
1972 Treating Children in Groups. San Francisco. Jossey-Boxx, Inc.

Rower, W. D., Jr., Amon, P. R. and Cramer, P. Understanding Intellectual Development. Hinsdale, Ill: The Dryden Press.

Sibbach, Lois and Jacobs, Alfred
Sequence Effects of Positive and Negative Personal Feedback Delivered to Mentally Retarded Participants in Cooperative Group Activity. (Unpublished manuscript)

Williams, J. L.
1973 Operant Learning: Procedure for changing behavior. Monterey, California: Brooks/Cole.

STUART FINE, M.B., F.R.C.P. (C) (Canada) and RUTH NASKE, M.D. (Austria)

PSYCHOSIS, PSYCHOSOMATIC ILLNESS AND CHRONIC ILLNESS IN CHILDREN

This workshop discussed separately the issues of childhood psychosis and those of psychosomatic and chronic physical illness.

CHILDHOOD PSYCHOSIS

It was maintained that the prognosis in childhood psychosis depended upon the child's testable intelligence, whether there were any organic factors, the ability to acquire language, and the rate at which any improvement was noted. Treatment methods included special education and language training; and medication was used only symptomatically. Many felt that psychoanalytically oriented psychotherapy had not been helpful.

In one series presented, only one in ten improved substantially, and in one in every six there had been a psychosocial stress that had precipitated the initial symptomatology and referral.

One resource person questioned whether the entity, psychosis in childhood, existed. He felt that many of the symptoms described could be understood if the relationship between parents and child were studied in detail, particularly the relationship between the father and child.

Another participant felt that there might be a lesion in the limbic system of the brain similar to that occurring in animals who had a poor orienting response.

Much discussion occurred about the provocative suggestion that this entity did not exist, and the majority of participants felt that this was a theoretical stance and that anyone who had been in clinical practice recognized that a clinical entity did exist and that the prognosis was guarded.

PSYCHOSOMATIC ILLNESS

The establishment of a separate psychiatric unit for children in a pediatric setting was felt to be an important development, particularly for children with psychosomatic illness. There were several dilemmas discussed, including the admission criteria for the psychiatric unit as opposed to a pediatric unit.

Several specific psychosomatic illnesses were discussed, particularly anorexia nervosa, where many felt that a combined psychoanalytically oriented psychotherapeutic approach given by the psychiatrist, and a firm medical approach given by the pediatrician, were effective methods of helping people suffering from this syndrome.

S. H. Fine, R. Krell, and Tsung-yi Lin (Eds.), 'Today's Priorities in Mental Health' 193–195.

The initial diagnosis of juvenile diabetes and the impact of traumatic head injury were both seen as crises for the child and his family, and the possibility of early intervention for both the child and his parents was presented as not only feasible but also important. The intervention in trichotillomania and alopecia areata was discussed, based on the presentation of one case history. Psychoanalytically oriented psychotherapy was recommended as the treatment of choice in cases with these troublesome symptoms. The effect of reducing stress on preschool children and the staff of preschoolers by adding personnel to day care centres, showed that conflicts between children, absenteeism in the staff, and anxiety in the children as measured by their catecholamine levels all diminished.

Theories to try to explain the development of psychosomatic illness in individuals were presented. One participant felt an imbalance between individual and social development resulted in psychosomatic illness, and a study on university students seemed to confirm that those students with psychosomatic illness did have this imbalance. The usefulness of Anna Freud's theories of development, particularly in early childhood, as they relate to oral, anal and locomotor areas, could be used to explain the development of psychosomatic illnesses.

Discussion centred around the syndrome of anorexia nervosa, and questions were raised as to whether there was an increasing incidence of this disease throughout the world. It was felt that perhaps in some South American countries there was in fact either no increase in incidence or it was not being recognized.

CHRONIC PHYSICAL DISABILITY

Educational approaches to children with cerebral palsy and autism were demonstrated by movies and the gain in skills was convincing. Consultation to specific wards in children's hospitals and specific programs such as burn units, renal dialysis units and intensive care units was mentioned. The reactions of children, parents and staff were examined, and methods of intervention were discussed.

SUMMARY

The focus of the workshop was the dissemination of ideas about etiology and treatment of children and adolescents with childhood psychosis, psychosomatic illness and chronic physical illness. Early and brief intervention were stressed as being very useful in the early stages of the development of psychosomatic illness and chronic physical illness. The importance of special education for childhood psychosis and the chronic physical illnesses was illustrated. Sharing of etiological theories about the onset of psychosomatic illness led to some interesting discussion.

RESOURCE PERSONS

Dr. J. Anderson (South Africa)
Dr. J. Breton (Canada)
Dr. M. Cederblad (Sweden)
Prof. C. Eggers (West Germany)
Mr. R. Fritz (USA)
Prof. I. Kolvin (UK)
Dr. E. Laible (Austria)
Dr. Y. Larsson (Sweden)
Dr. E. Marini (Italy)
Dr. E. Mitrani (Israel)
Dr. Ch. Mussert (Holland)
Dr. R. Navon (Israel)
Dr. W. Pieringer (Austria)
Prof. Q. Rae-Grant (Canada)
Dr. V. Sanua (USA)
Dr. J. Van Leeuwen (Canada)
Dr. R. Zimin (Israel)

EUGENE B. BRODY, M.D. (U.S.A.), N. KAPOR-STANULOVIC, Ph.D. (Yugoslavia), D. DEANE (Switzerland) and BENJAMIN VIEL, M.D. (U.K.)

MAKING UNWANTED CHILDREN WANTED: PREPARATION FOR PARENTHOOD

The United States Joint Commission on the Mental Health of Children has defined the rights of infants. Among these are the rights to be wanted, to be born healthy, to live in a healthy environment, to obtain satisfaction of basic needs, to receive continuous loving care, to acquire the intellectual and emotional skills necessary to achieve individual aspirations, and to cope effectively in society. It is clear that such fundamental rights are a prescription for mental health and should be included in all mental health programmes.

Upon quick review of the conditions of the child in the present world, it is easy to conclude that such rights are far from being implemented. Even in the 'developed' world, there are laws that are clearly in opposition to several of the above rights. For example, in the U.S., restriction of Federal funds for abortion is responsible for a great number of children being born unwanted. This is true particularly among the poor. Those born unwanted have less of a chance to obtain the right to continuous loving care or the satisfaction of basic needs. It is unlikely that we shall have a healthy society when a great number of individuals are born under conditions that would make them violent and resentful.

In the 'underdeveloped' world the situation is much worse, not only because the countries are poorer, but because the number of those born unwanted, owing to present legislation, is much greater. For example, it is estimated that the number of deprived or abandoned children in Brazil is 25 million. No doubt similar figures could be obtained in other Latin American countries as well as in the rest of the underdeveloped world.

It was the consensus of the group that it is the duty of mental health workers to join the fight for the removal of the present barriers that prevent implementation of fundamental rights. Mental health workers are directly concerned with the reduction of unwanted births as well as the timing, spacing and total number of children born to a woman, as these affect psychological well-being.

To reduce unwanted births it is essential that all vulnerable people have a clear understanding of the methods to regulate fertility as well as easy access to services. Mental health programmes have in this respect two sets of concerns. One is to help parents to regulate their own fertility (family planning), the other to help them to become more adequate parents for the children they already have (family life).

Even in societies in which contraceptive methods are available and easily obtainable, unwanted pregnancies occur, owing to non-use of contraceptives,

S. H. Fine, R. Krell, and Tsung-yi Lin (Eds.), 'Today's Priorities in Mental Health' 197–201.

failure of the method used, or to human error in the way they are being used. Especially among the young, now living in a much more liberated society, unwanted pregnancies are reaching epidemic proportions. In the face of such evidence the group discussed abortion, the only method of avoiding an unwanted birth once pregnancy has begun.

Today abortion is legal in many countries, the great majority of them being in the developed world. In others, it is illegal even to save the life of the mother, to prevent the birth of a sick child, or to prevent birth due to rape or incestuous sexual relations. No doubt where it is illegal it is also widely practised very safely when performed by professionals. However, this service is often exclusively available to those able to pay. It is an extremely dangerous procedure when performed by unskilled abortionists. Thirty percent of the obstetric beds in Brazilian hospitals are occupied by women who have had complications of illegal abortion performed outside hospital. A conservative estimate would be that 6 million illegal abortions are performed yearly in the Latin American countries. Acceptance of abortion depends on the different interpretation that each society has about when life begins. This interpretation has varied throughout history. For some it starts with the fecundation of the ovum, for others at the moment of implantation, for others at birth, and there are even societies in which real life is considered to begin after birth when the child has proven its ability to survive in the external environment. In the absence of a common biological definition, the beginning of life is defined by social interpretation.

As in many groups that discuss abortion, the question of the influence of the Catholic church was paramount. From the discussions it was clear that the strong opposition to abortion on the part of the Catholic church was mainly influencing governments rather than populations. Governments fear a confrontation with the hierarchy of the church. However, 80% of those hospitalized for complications resulting from illegal abortion in the Latin American countries declare that they are Catholic. In the State of Rhode Island, a predominantly Catholic community, 65% of the women requesting legal abortion identified themselves as being Catholic.

Using infant mortality as an indication of the existence of possible rejection by the mother, in Chile mothers under 20 or over 35 show a much higher rate of infant mortality. Regardless of age, infant mortality increases with parity over three. It is claimed that to diminish infant mortality without diminishing great multiparity and pregnancies at adverse ages would be impossible.

In the absence of physical signs at birth that show decreased biological capacity for survival, it is suggested that the higher infant mortality reported is due to an unsuitable environment provided by the mother. Such an adverse environment is not always owing to poverty. It is quite possible that higher infant mortality among great multiparae or mothers who are too young is due to a form of unconscious infanticide. It may well happen that the mother sees a partial solution to her problem if the child dies. However, more research is necessary before this can be concluded. If this is proved, it was suggested that the present education of the younger generation is based on a misguided understanding that all women have a similar degree of maternal instinct. It may well be that there are women who do not wish ever to be mothers. A more sincere educational approach should teach the young that it is not a duty to have children but it is a duty to have healthy children.

Death is certainly only the tip of the iceberg. There are conditions which cause a great number of physical and psychological traumas (undernourishment, deprivation of love, deprivation of stimulation, child abuse, etc.).

Other papers indicated the importance of psychological factors in mother and child relationships, including the ambivalent feelings of the mother, especially when pregnant for the first time. Unresolved tensions may induce problems that have great importance and that should be prevented since they may influence future mother/child relationships. There is evidence that the proper treatment of recognizable anxieties during pregnancy prevents difficulties and complications during delivery and facilitates future normal relationships within the family.

It is incorrect to consider that pregnancy and delivery are the responsibility of the mother and do not concern the male partner. Group courses for couples have proven to be a great help in dealing with emotional tensions and give the couple a sense of common responsibility. It was reported that when the male partner is present during the delivery it increases the joint feeling of responsibility and also prolongs the period of lactation. This is a good indication that the amount of milk a mother has depends a great deal on psychological factors.

Research shows that breast-feeding is more successfully accomplished and lasts for a longer period of time when earlier skin contact between the mother and the newborn occurs. This has psychological implications as well as practical implications in attempting to increase the present small number of mothers who breast-feed.

When the world is observing signs of rejection of children, it is logical that means to prevent this should be developed. A description of the efforts being carried out in this regard in the United Kingdom through a team of general practitioners, midwives, health nurses and social workers was described. It was said that the work began before birth with visits during the prenatal period as well as after the birth and during the early period of the life of the child, later the health nurse, and later still the school nurse. From the early visits nurses could identify risk, and through the subsequent visits they would be able to educate the mother and direct high risk cases to special institutions. Since acceptance of this service is a voluntary act on the part of the family it is possible that those who do not accept the services offered are those most at risk. The description of this work gave rise to many questions about the training of visiting personnel, the referral systems, the present coverage and the delegation of responsibility. There was a feeling that no matter how good a service of this sort could be, it could not be applied in the underdeveloped world, chiefly owing to cost and the lack of trained personnel.

A strong appeal was made to promote male participation in contraceptive use. Work carried out in the City of San Francisco was described.

It has been claimed that the decline in the birth rate that began 100 years ago in what today are industrial societies, was achieved with a great deal of male cooperation (coitus interruptus). The availability of female contraceptives has created a disproportion in the responsibilities of the partners. Males now tend to think that contraception is the responsibility of the women. Great efforts should be made to change such an attitude.

All the papers presented at this workshop moved the group to present a resolution to the Executive Committee of the World Federation for Mental Health.

RESOLUTION FROM WORKSHOP NO. 14 'MAKING UNWANTED CHILDREN WANTED'

TO: Executive Committee, WFMH

The Federation therefore resolves that:
These rights are fundamental to the mental health of parents and children, and should be a concern of all mental health and psychiatric programs.

In order to ensure the rights of children and parents and particularly to reduce the number of unwanted, neglected, abused or abandoned children, and to enhance responsible and effective parenthood, the Federation proposes that the following items should be part of the action programs of all volunteer, professional, private and governmental, mental health and psychiatric organizations and institutions, and of all other health, educational or welfare-related organizations and institutions concerned with the well-being of parents, infants, children and adolescents:

1. Family life and sex education, including attention to love, intimate communication, and the relation of sexuality to reproduction for all children, and adults, using the schools and other educational and informational institutions.

2. Education for such programs in all curricula for students, professionals and volunteers concerned with children and parenthood, including training for law, education and social welfare, as well as health and related human service fields.

3. Family planning information and services for both men and women in all countries and cultures.

4. Special counselling for parents and children at risk for impaired mental health or psychiatric disturbance, and in particular for psychologically or psychiatrically handicapped men and women of reproductive age.

5. Equal access to high quality reproductive health care for all people who want and require it including consultation for and implementation of pregnancy-termination or sterilization.

6. That concerned professional and voluntary organizations monitor the legal-judicial structure and social circumstances of their own and other countries in order to understand the contexts in which individuals and couples relate sexually, reproduce and rear children; to exert public pressure aimed at modifying policies which impede reproductive health and diminish the rights of children; introduce policies which guarantee them; and promote research, education and services relevant to making all births intended and all children wanted.

RESOURCE PERSONS

Helio Aguinaga (Brazil)
Susan Bram (USA)
Zdenek Dytrich (Czechoslovakia)
Stephen Fleck (USA)
Lucile Newman (USA)
Sallye B. Petersen (USA)

JOHN DOWNING, Ph.D. (Canada), IRA GROSS, Ph.D. (U.S.A.),
ADMA d'HEURLE, Ph.D. (U.S.A.)

HEALTHY ATTITUDES TOWARD DEVELOPING MASCULINE AND FEMININE ROLES

SUMMARY STATEMENT

The focus of the wide-ranging discussion throughout the workshop was the underlying concern, expressed by most of the participants, of how can the study of sex role expectations, attitudes and behaviors contribute to the development of healthy males and females. There was general agreement that the prevailing biases constrain the development of healthy and creative persons who are free to actualize their full individual potential. The essential contradictions between affiliative and achievement needs, expressive and instrumental functions, and private and public spheres of experience that exist in the stereotypic definition of masculinity and femininity were generally recognized as serious impediments to mental health.

The different treatment of the sexes in early childhood and throughout the elementary school years was discussed. The ways in which young boys and girls (preschool) differ in their interactions with the environment were touched on through summaries of the research literature and new empirical studies. The school as an increasingly powerful agent in the socialization process received a great deal of attention. Different aspects of the school culture were examined with particular emphasis on their effect on the perpetuation of sex role stereotypes as well as their potential for bringing about change in the prevailing value system. Curricular materials, methods of instruction, school organization and management as well as the school's hidden curriculum were recognized as a means of influencing children's understanding of the meaning of their gender identity, their feelings about this identity and the behaviors that are congruent with it.

Studies of differential patterns of academic achievement, of aspirations and achievement motivations and of modes of peer interaction were reported and discussed.

The school's potential to correct the biases that exist in sex role definitions was recognized and some of the means by which this potential could be realized were explored. Particular attention was given to the curriculum. Non-sexist educational materials were presented and discussed. The value of introducing such materials into the schools was recognized, but not without due appreciation that the non-sexist nature of curricular materials is only one of the many important criteria of an educationally sound curriculum.

S. H. Fine, R. Krell, and Tsung-yi Lin (Eds.), 'Today's Priorities in Mental Health' 203–205.

The nurture of an atmosphere in the school that would facilitate an open dialogue with boys and girls as well as educators and parents regarding differences and similarities in sex role behaviors was seen as an essential element in any attempt to effect change in the status quo. Particular means for initiating and sustaining a meaningful dialogue were given some consideration. Recent legislation, for example, was indicated as one of the measures that has been found effective in stimulating fruitful discussions in many schools and community contexts.

Along with the high expectations for the possibilities of change through the school, there was an expression of true appreciation of the many demands that are increasingly made upon the school in modern technological societies.

Role perceptions of adult men and women were discussed. Particular emphasis was given to the role of language and specific suggestions were put forth for sharpening sensitivity to exclusionary language and finding ways to eliminate it without undue hindrance to effective communication. The effects of adult role perception on reproduction, family patterns and occupational activity were considered. Some apprehension was expressed about the acceptance of non-traditional ways of defining the place of reproduction and of parenting in human experience. However, the majority of opinions supported the recognition of and support for alternative modalities to the extent that they recognize the value of the individual human being and extend the margin of the person's freedom of choice. Defining the responsibility for the care of children was seen as a primary task in any society, and it was understood that this responsibility will be carried out by committed and eminently qualified people.

Considerable time was devoted to discussing the place of the scientific study of sex differences and the opinions here tended to be divergent. Some workshop members felt that scientific evidence about sex differences is the only valid basis for any discussion of policies and programs affecting the lives of males and females. Others felt that the scientific study of sex differences to date has put inordinate weight on the differences and not given enough consideration to the congruencies and similarities between the sexes. Many agreed that the discussion of child caring methods, educational programs and other humane practices must proceed in the light of what is already known about the socialization process and that this must be done with due regard for the cultural context.

As deliberation proceeded the members of the workshop became convinced of the value of the continuation of our work through future workshops in an effort to (1) deepen our own understanding of the theme and its ramifications and (2) help us actualize our collective desire to communicate the insights and understandings gained from this experience to a wider audience.

As a group the members of the workshop became more firmly committed to working actively towards the goal of equality between the sexes in our role as mental health professionals, in educational institutions, health care delivery systems and in the community. In this capacity we recognize that we can promote mental health through:

(1) Setting standards
(2) Acting as role models
(3) Changing and shaping attitudes
(4) Enhancing equal opportunities for both sexes
(5) Promoting a humanistic dialogue regarding sex roles

RECOMMENDATIONS

The consensus of the workshop was to:

(1) Continue the work begun in 1977 with the first workshop on "sex-role attitudes at the crossroads" at the World Congress of Mental Health, Vancouver, Canada, through future workshops at WFMH conferences.

(2) Assess and examine the definitions, attitudes and behaviors of mental health professionals in regard to sex roles, by way of:

(a) A variety of collaborative cross-cultural research projects, and
(b) A survey (mailed questionnaire) of the World Federation for Mental Health membership on sex-role attitudes (a summary of this survey to be presented at the next Congress), and
(c) Monitoring and improving our own organizational activities, e.g. through use of non-sexist language in conference program materials and avoidance of presumptious terms such as 'ladies' programs' for spouses and accompanying guests, disproportionate selection of males as invited keynote speakers, and sexist bias in some of the presentations.

(3) Urge that the World Federation for Mental Health exhort mental health professionals to raise to conscious awareness the dangers to mental health of sex-role stereotyping, and in the process, to examine their own attitudes.

RESOURCE PERSONS

Cheryl Benard (Austria)
Susan Bram (USA)
J. Cohen (USA)
Charles Downing (UK)
John Downing (Canada)
Carol Dwyer (USA)
Shirley B. Ernest (USA)
Alice Gross (USA)
Mahesh Gupta (Austria)
Selma Hughes (USA)
Corinne Hutt (UK)
I. Kallab (Lebanon)
Betty Kleiman (Canada)
Sophia Leung (Canada)
I. Lorfing (Lebanon)
J. Abu Nasr (Lebanon)
Pirkko Niemla (Finland)
Rama S. Pandey (USA)
Edit Schlaffer (Austria)
Denis Chimaeze Ugwuegbu (Nigeria)
V. Widmark-Petersson (USA)

L. Y. RABKIN, Ph.D. (U.S.A.), P. KOMLOSI, Ph.D. (Hungary), and
R. KRELL, M.D., F.R.C.P. (C) (Canada)

PSYCHOTHERAPY OF THE WHOLE FAMILY

The aim of this workshop was to provide a cross-cultural perspective on the current state of family therapy, its theoretical basis, methodology, and general and specific applications. The nine papers presented examined aspects of family therapy in six countries. Comments and responses from participants further broadened the range of participation.

Family therapy is to be differentiated from the more inclusive term 'family assessment'. Whatever the form of distress and disturbance in a family, assessment must be made in several areas before treatment is begun. These include a system-oriented diagnosis of family conflicts, strengths, values, and motivations, an evaluation of the family members' understanding of their roles in the difficulties of the identified patient, an estimation of the effects that intervention in the family system may have, and a global evaluation of how the family works as a group.

Diagnosis of the family's central conflicts provides information necessary for effective intervention, whether this is to be in the form of family group therapy or some method of individual psychotherapy. In the latter case, the therapist will better be able to recognize how family conflicts are reflected in the individual patient's functioning and difficulties experienced in living.

The indications for family therapy are several. When the term 'family therapy' is used, as a synonym for a general orientation towards working with a family system, then 'family therapy' is a necessity in all cases of distress. However, this need not include all family members at the same time.

When family therapy is used as a term for a therapeutic procedure involving the whole family, there are a number of prerequisites: (1) the therapist undertaking the task must be trained in some form of this procedure or be under the supervision of a trained professional; (2) the family members must give their informed consent to the planned intervention; (3) the family must agree to be engaged in the process. There are many formulations of the universal parameters of the family. These include the family as: mediator between the child and society, transmitter of cultural values, teacher of methods to carry out tasks, orientator to goals, transmitter and assigner of power, teacher of responsibility and effective regulation. In addition, it is a primary source for the development of individual and group sense of self as well as a vehicle for learning modes of communication. These various parameters can be partly summarized in five categories: tasks and goals, boundary maintenance, leadership, regulation of effectivity, and communication.

S. H. Fine, R. Krell, and Tsung-yi Lin (Eds.), 'Today's Priorities in Mental Health' 207–209.

The problems which arise in families are manifold, but these are generally conflicts concerning how different family members feel, believe, think or act. Because the family is a system, the ways such conflicts are expressed and perpetuated involve the participation of all its members. There are various terms in the field of family therapy which attempt to define some of these family patterns: e.g., triangulation, complementarity and symmetry, and cross-generational coalitions. The general roles of the family therapist are fourfold. First, the family therapist acts as a *mediator* of family conflicts. Second, he/she is an *educator*, teaching methods of conflict resolution and the workings of the family system. Third, he/she is a translator of the misunderstood language of different generations, of society's expectations and rules, and of the symptomatic behavior of the family into understandable words; and fourth, he/she is a spokesperson, sometimes for one member or side in a family, at other times for the family *to* society or for society *to* the family. The specific methods used by family therapists in carrying out these roles, include the clarification and interpretation of family patterns of communication and role allocations, the use of paradoxical behavior prescription to induce a change in the family system which maintains the symptomatology of one of its members, the modelling of behavior, role playing, and the induction of family crises to disrupt destructive cycles of behavior.

In the United States, where family therapy has experienced much of its twenty-five year growth, there has been a proliferation of its techniques. There has also been a commitment to careful evaluation of the effectiveness of family therapy. Although the literature on outcome has been equivocal, a recent survey of studies suggests that family therapy is, indeed, quite effective as a treatment modality. It appears to be in use in all areas of the country; in hospitals, clinics, and in independent practice. There has also been much teaching of family systems theory and family therapy techniques outside traditional mental health settings, for example in Departments of Family Medicine and Pediatrics.

Family therapy is a relatively new technique in Europe. It has been accepted with great enthusiasm by a few practitioners in such countries as the United Kingdom, Switzerland, Greece and Hungary. This is true, as well, in Mexico, Israel, Canada, Australia and New Zealand. It is being used as a treatment modality in psychiatric hospitals, child guidance clinics, sports medicine clinics, adult out-patient departments, and psychosomatic medicine programs.

There is a concern on the part of therapists everywhere about the special problems of countertransference in family therapy. The intensity of interaction between therapist and family facilitates the arousal in the therapist of unresolved issues of his/her own family and may provoke a variety of distortions in the therapist's perceptions, feelings and actions. To help control such phenomena, it is important that the therapist have adequate training and supervision. The ethical issues involving the problem of privacy in family therapy must also be carefully investigated and considered.

Cross-cultural investigations of family system variables and therapy outcome will help to clarify much that remains obscure in the process of symptom formation and the effectiveness of different techniques. It is hoped that the group of participants in this workshop will attempt to facilitate such cross-cultural investigations, and share further results and experiences at the next WFMH Congress in 1981.

RESOURCE PERSONS

Dr. Evangelos Dimitriou (Greece)
Dr. Stephen Fleck (USA)
Dr. Raymundo Macias (Mexico)
Dr. Antonia Sidorowicz (USA)
Dr. A. Wille (Switzerland)
Dr. Alexander Zaphiris (USA)

I. LEE GISLASON, M.D., F.R.C.P. (C) (U.S.A.), Prof. Dr H. LECHNER (Austria), ESTELLE STEVENS, M.D., F.R.C.P. (C) (Canada)

THE INFLUENCE OF MASS MEDIA (TELEVISION) ON CHILDREN – PROSOCIAL ASPECTS

Television has appeared as a new family member and second teacher in the home. Its influence is powerful and persuasive, transcending literacy and demography. Television operates as a major agent of socialization, with preemptive powers over the growing child's range of attention and activities. By the time the average American child has reached the high school age of 15, he has spent more hours in television viewing than in the classroom.

This workshop was a continuation of the 1977 Workshop on Influence of Mass Media on Children and differed in that it focused primarily on the prosocial aspects of television.

The question 'What is prosocial television?' was discussed by workshop participants and opinions varied with the philosophy of each country represented. An attempt to deliniate a definition of prosocial television which could apply to all countries was made. Traditionally, a prosocial television has referred to programs which were designed to influence viewers in a 'positive' way. This involves a value judgement and usually refers to both psychological and behavioral influences. On the psychological level, prosocial television should enhance a viewer's feelings of self-worth, confidence and ability to deal with an ever-increasingly complex world; on the behavioral level, it should enhance a viewer's repertoire of actions and skills which permit effective interaction with others and his environment.

Criteria which can be used in judging whether a viewer will profit from his contact with television are:

1. Does the television experience expand how we learn? Does it give us the cognitive skills, the curiosity and behaviors through which we seek greater knowledge and understanding so that we can continue to mature as individuals and members of society?
2. Does the television experience increase knowledge?
3. Does the television experience expand our repertoire of behavioral and social skills necessary in dealing with one another?
4. Does the television experience expand our repertoire of emotional experience and skills? Can we learn to be more spontaneous in our displays of friendliness and humor, or learn to delay immediate gratification and be more persistent?

In our discussion of how television and radio are used in different countries it was apparent that patterns of production and viewing vary significantly.

S. H. Fine, R. Krell, and Tsung-yi Lin (Eds.), 'Today's Priorities in Mental Health' 211–213.

Although the workshop was designed originally to focus on prosocial aspects of mass media, workshop participants and resource persons introduced a wide range of ideas.

There was major concern about who controlled the media. Is it the child, parent, community, producer or government? For example, in some countries the media is designed with the education of the child as a primary goal and the programs are without advertisements and funded by the Government. In other countries profit is the primary consideration in programming, consequently, entertainment of the child is a primary goal with advertisements as the source of revenue. It is clear that control is different in each system, and that each has merits and potentials for misuse.

Programs produced in some countries are exported to others by circumstance (being geographical neighbors), or intent (sale of prerecorded programs). It was suggested that we are progressing toward a 'Global Village'. Countries can learn about each other; however, there is understandable concern by lesser developed, importing countries that programs from more developed countries will eventually jeopardize their culture and values.

New technologies, such as satelite television, videorecorders, 80 channel availability and computer terminals attached to television monitors are changing the media. It was suggested that within a few years children rather than being the passive recipients of a small number of centrally produced program channels, will be the active consumers of a wide variety of media choices. How is this possible? The cost of the complex technology is decreasing rapidly, parallelling the revolution in computer technology. It was pointed out in one study that children watched 20–25 hours of television per week whether they had one or four televisions channels available. It is anticipated that with an availability of, for example, 80 channels, viewing time per week will not increase although the opportunities for prosocial television viewing will be enhanced.

There was agreement that advertising to children under 8 years of age is undesirable, as they are not able to evaluate the material presented to them.

Concern was expressed by participants from all countries about the amount of television designed for adults that is watched by children. In many situations these programs are not appropriate for young children and should be carefully monitored.

Responsibility for what a child views and implementing constructive change lies with the parent, producer and government. Education regarding children's programming was advocated.

In order to provide a framework to develop constructive use of television, guidelines for selecting programming for children were presented:

1. Does the program appeal to the audience for whom intended? (A program for 12-year olds should be different from a program for 6-year olds.)

2. Does the program present racial groups positively and does it show them

in situations that enhance the self-image of children from different countries? (Who has the lead roles? Who is the professional or leader and who is the villain?)

3. Does the program present gender roles and adult roles positively? (Are the men either super-heroes or incompetents? Are the women flighty and disposed to chicanery? Are teenagers portrayed with adult characteristics?)

4. Does the program present social issues that are appropriate for the child viewer and perhaps are something a child can act on at a child's level? (Litter versus atomic fallout, or pet care versus saving wolves.)

5. Does the program encourage worthwhile ideals, values and beliefs?

6. Does the program present conflict that a child can understand and does it demonstrate positive techniques for resolving the conflict?

7. Does the program stimulate constructive activities and does it enhance the quality of a child's play?

8. Does the program separate fact from fantasy? Does it separate advertisements from program content?

9. Does the program present humor at a child's level? (Or is it adult sarcasm, ridicule or an adult remembering what he thought was funny from his childhood?)

10. Does the program have a pace that allows the child to absorb and contemplate the material presented?

11. Does the program have artistic qualities?

12. Has your child seen an appropriate amount of television for the day? (Or is it time to turn off the set?)

Television is here to stay. It has progressed through its own childhood stage and is in its passage through adolescence. Television may eventually become a mature adult. However, it remains a complicated innovation and an institution of uncertain potential.

RESOURCE PERSONS

Gregory T. Fouts (Canada)
Monika Henreid (USA)
Aletha Huston Stein (USA)
Hans-Jorg Tinchon (Austria)
Toshio Watanabe (Japan)
Sally Williams (USA)
Tannis MacBeth Williams (Canada)
John Wright (USA)

R. L. BEISER, M.Ed. (Canada), D. S. BUTT, Ph.D. (Canada), and
G. MORRIS CARSTAIRS, M.D. (UK)

CREATIVE LEISURE FOR CHILDREN AND FAMILIES

The origin of this workshop, 'Creative Leisure for Children and Families' is traceable to the World Federation for Mental Health Congress held in Vancouver, B.C., August 1977. At that time, the late Dr. Margaret Mead participated in a discussion on the importance of leisure and suggested that a conference focusing on the subject be held in the future. Her concerns were shared by several Japanese colleagues who were also in attendance and who subsequently organized the Tsukuba Conference in late 1978. It was most unfortunate that Dr. Mead did not live to attend what was a truly interdisciplinary experience. Representatives from academia, government and business gathered for a memorable time of planning for the future on the theme, 'Toward the Social System of the 21st Century: Free Time and Quality of Life'. The present workshop grew out of the Tsukuba experience and is a continuation of that look into the future. In it one finds the extension of a relatively new idea; that leisure is important in the future development and well-being of humankind.

Changing values in the world, freedom of choice and the implications of each for the future, were the themes emerging from workshop proceedings. In summarizing, we shall divert slightly from the actual order of presentations to discuss the content of papers and commentaries under three headings: 1. definitions; 2. the role of creativity in mental health and 3. redirections in value orientations.

1. DEFINITIONS AND DIRECTIONS

'Yutori' is the Japanese concept referring to a mental attitude embracing that which is not a dire necessity. It is a quality of not being tightly structured or a condition in which energy is available to a person or thing in excess of everyday demands. This creative energy may be used to describe a person in a work situation whose competence and control allow him or her to be somewhat detached and to extend in spirit beyond the demands of everyday duties. It is a 'latitude of mind' which gives one room in oneself to look at other things. This concept formed a base for what would follow.

Leisure is best defined as a psychological attitude involving freedom and intrinsic motivation. Both are basic to mental health. There are no external constraints to a state of leisure which is experienced for its own sake and should not be confused with the American definition of creativity in which a product is involved. This was the direction suggested by an American psychologist who

S. H. Fine, R. Krell, and Tsung-yi Lin (Eds.), 'Today's Priorities in Mental Health' 215–218.

concluded with a description of a differential typology between job, work and leisure.

In planning for the new freedom to be showered on a large part of the population with the technological development expected in the 21st century, a Japanese colleague suggested that release, recreation and disciplined leisure (here taken to mean selected, *self*-imposed) are best differentiated. The first can become self-destructive as in release through drugs or alcohol. The second can also exhaust. It includes the great interest in physical recreation which mushroomed with the industrial revolution when a 'leisured class' emerged. The third brings psychological security and aesthetic experience. It is the third which we should pursue because one can never tire of disciplined leisure. Both release and recreation may tire and exhaust, but disciplined leisure embraces and reflects the cultivated life.

2. THE IMPORTANCE OF 'CREATIVE' LEISURE

The majority of papers, and perhaps the major substance of the workshop, had to do with reports of what people were doing throughout the world to encourage self-expressions and free choice in various situations and in various groups of people. We follow with a summary of these ideas and reports.

Village India was contrasted with westernized India. In village life it is not necessary to programme leisure and play activities. They are already an integral part of everyday life. Thus storytellers are a popular feature and convey religious, moral and adventure themes to the population. Village dramas are also embedded in social life as is the play of children. In contrast to westernized ways, toys are not featured. The young Indian child would not, for example, play with dolls as real babies would be plentiful in village life and in need of attention. Various releases are apparent which afford opportunities for segments of the population to express hostilities to others, through enactments, on special occasions. An example would be a song sung by a group with a somewhat sarcastic theme. The importance of the movie house in transmitting cultural values and religious themes in the cities was also pointed out.

Our presenter from Brazil argued against the notion that attention to leisure in developing groups is too expensive and a mere trifle. She stated that leisure education is worth all funds invested because the constructive use of leisure time can aid healthful development by teaching freedom of choice and allowing people to cope with a changing environment. Education in leisure is education against dependency and perhaps even against poverty. We must try to divert persons away from the concept of 'killing time' and toward the concept of using time for personal expression, human growth and the exploration of self.

Czechoslovakian immigrants to the City of Calgary, Alberta, were participants in the study done at the University of Alberta, Calgary, Canada. Methods adopted by immigrants, in order to cope with and adjust to a foreign environment, were documented. A new language, an emphasis on outdoor activity and a nuclear family orientation had to be adopted to a background which featured another language, an emphasis upon artistic-cultural activities and a relative independence of family members during free time. The people developed what was described as a dual identity, participating gradually in the life and activities of their new home yet strengthening their family ties and family activities in order to preserve something of the old. These adjustments enabled immigrants to maintain a mental balance between their old and new environments.

The importance of freedom of expression in visual arts, song, dance and drama were described in an Ontario, Canada school for the disadvantaged. Growth through common vehicles of communication was stressed. This theme was continued in a song, 'Home in Your Heart', which the presenters had composed and arranged in celebration of the International Year of the Child. It was sung at the request of workshop members who much appreciated this unique contribution.

From Israel we were presented with a theory out of which has grown a method for dealing with the social problems of a people who are under pressure to change. The social pressures released by rapid industrialization and automation were described as they affect people who have reached middle class status. With the assumption that persons are born creative, the goals adopted for community and personal growth are: 1. for people to define their needs; 2. for people to define the resources of the community and 3. for people to bring the needs and the resources together in the service of development and problem resolutions. The techniques in practice begin by encouraging persons to be creative and to provide descriptions of their problems and probable solutions through their enactment in drama and storytelling. A group worker and an artisan typically work together in encouraging this creative and practical expression with the purpose of fostering creative growth and creative solutions to personal and social problems.

3. REDIRECTIONS IN VALUE ORIENTATIONS

Three papers examined some of the changing values in the modern world and proposed new directions. One from Japan called for a strengthening of family ties and values in that the family is the first and most important socializing agent of future world citizens. Two changes in direction were proposed. On the one hand there was a call for more self-insight and individual responsibility by knowing oneself through self-reflection. Secondly, it was noted that the traditional role of women in technological society had, in a sense, been undermined. In the future that same role could become a role of increased leadership and self-fulfillment (as it has been in the past and continues to be for many). With the change from working for remuneration in technological societies to the new theme of using one's time creatively and constructively for the betterment of all without remuneration . . . the traditional role of women may reach a new significance as a constructive example to others.

From the approach of systems analysis, the relationships between world stabilization and increased leisure time were described. Another of our colleagues from Japan documented the great amount of 'free time' awaiting persons, not only during their retirement, but also in younger years as a result of motorization, computerization and automation. To compensate for the decreased demands on special functions with the arrival of each technology; (1) sport and recreation, (2) liberal arts and (3) crafts and survival arts have risen respectively to fill the voids. All call for the development and practice of disciplined leisure in the future.

Finally, the competitive ethic in North America, as reflected in sport organization for young children, was criticized as being personally and socially destructive. A competence model of children's play and leisure activity was proposed as an alternative in which the individual is encouraged to participate for intrinsic reward and for the pleasure of skill development and the growth of both self-esteem and self-confidence. It was proposed that a competence orientation would lead to feelings of social cooperation and to the motivation to seek creative solutions to later challenges in personal, social and political life. These recommendations were based upon studies of the child and the psychology of sport in Canada.

In summary, there were several common premises in the papers presented, the most basic of which was a belief in the capacity of the individual to develop constructively and to build a better world if that individual is given freedom of choice and the opportunity to create. Mental health and constructive living will emerge from the creative, free and experimental use of leisure.

RESOURCE PERSONS

Takeo L. Doi (Japan)
John Neulinger (USA)
Yoshiko Nomura (Japan)
Shoichi Watanabe (Japan)
Ethel Bauzer Madeiros (Brazil)
Jarmila L. A. Horna (Canada)
Louis Miller (Israel)
Yoshiyuki Matsuda (Japan)
Yana Vlcek (Canada)
Janine G. Schott (Canada)

SOPHIA LEUNG, M.S.W (Canada), MEI-CHEN LIN, M.S.W (Canada), LYNN CARTER, M.S.W (Canada), A.K. de VRIES (Holland)

MENTAL HEALTH AND SCHOOL

Schools may affect the mental health of children and their families in a number of different ways: they may act as a setting for preventive mental health activities; they may act as a source of mental health problems; they may provide help for troubled children and their families. When a child experiences school failure, it is most important to examine the school and family conditions rather than being too quick to label the child as the problem.

While the themes expressed above reflect universal concerns, specific subthemes emerge, according to the culture and context in which schools are assessed. Japanese pre-school children need to learn cooperative behavior, to try accommodative social solutions with peers when they are confronted with aggression and competition. In order to foster the development of initiative and individuality among preschoolers, schools must provide solitary play opportunities and small-group experiences. In Taiwan, elementary school boys experience more pressure and stresses than girls due to high parental expectation, sex stereotyping of the male child and the limited resources and physical facilities at school. A flexible and growth-oriented educational approach for Taiwan boys may induce better adjustment. Two thirds of Austrian children have been found to experience school difficulties and behavior problems due to academic pressure and competition. In the Netherlands, a special training program of 'positive discrimination' was given to the teachers of kindergartens and elementary schools. The positive approaches enhanced the teacher's attitudes and approaches to the young children. In British Columbia, Canada, it is interesting to note that many adolescents with behavior problems have a concurrent learning disability. These adolescents all require alternative or remedial educational assistance combined with therapeutic help as integral parts of their treatment. It was found that Canadian children with a syndrome of constitutionally short stature, delayed puberty and obesity suffered from personality disturbance based on poor body image. They also exhibited neurotic symptoms of anxiety, aggression, depression and poor peer relationships. These children also experienced school problems, academic underachievement and learning difficulties.

Selection pressures and the demands for academic performance make the college students particularly vulnerable to depression, suicide and serious psychiatric disorders. The students' suicide rates in highly esteemed universities like Oxford and Cambridge are higher than the suicide rates for students in other, more average universities. In Hong Kong, socio-cultural factors which influence the mental health of the university students include cultural values

S. H. Fine, R. Krell, and Tsung-yi Lin (Eds.), 'Today's Priorities in Mental Health' 219–221.

relating to the sick role, family attitudes towards authority and discipline, individual suppression of sexuality, the changing role of women and changing family patterns. About 1–2% of Hong Kong University students are affected by serious psychiatric disorder; a further 10–15% suffer from emotional impairment. In Japan, college students are also facing academic competition and social pressure to succeed. It seems that the existing student health services are highly inadequate on most university campuses. A need exists for helping services based on a positive approach which will not force students into patient roles.

In the area of community and adult education, various developments are occurring in different countries. In the United Kingdom, community educational projects have been developed to provide support and practical services to isolated and needy parents. Three innovative programmes in this area include: locally financed nursery centre facilities which provide learning experiences for young mothers and their children in a poor housing community; parents and children's projects aimed at reducing illiteracy; and a national parent education scheme which encourages parents' initiative, self-reliance, and interest in their children's development and education. In Western Canada, 'Family Life Education' programs provide parents basic information and learning experience in child development and management through group discussion and professional counselling. Parents may learn effective parenting techniques and a better understanding of their child's education and needs.

In the United States, recent legislation assures the provision of education for all handicapped children. Special programs for the handicapped utilizing the concept of 'least restrictive environment' and mainstreaming (placing handicapped and non-handicapped children together in classrooms) have been widely adopted. However, it is essential to develop creative approaches and procedures to make the learning experience of the handicapped a true entry into the normal world.

In comparing East and West, developing and developed countries, the following points can be made. Although many mental hygiene needs are common to developed and developing countries, the issue pre-eminent in many developing countries is providing adequate education. The role of the family system appears to be different in the East and West. In the East, the stable family seems to impose a cost to individualism and self-actualization. In the West, the demise of the stable family has occurred at the price of increased loneliness for the individual. Nevertheless, the need to improve educational systems in all countries, the need to minimize the stress engendered by extraordinary examinations and the need to encourage the development of the positive aspects within the school system are universal and essential for all children and families in the world.

RESOURCE PERSONS

Ernst Bergen (Austria)
Donna O'Connell Blatt (USA)
Walter Rind (Austria)
Tsune Shirai (Japan)

James Carter (Canada)
Carola Eisenberg (USA)
Leon Eisenberg (USA)
Max H. Friedrich (Austria)
E. J. Goodacre (UK)
G. Lyketsos (Greece)
D. J. Pallis (Greece)
Freya W. Owen (USA)
Karam Singer (Hong Kong)
Wei-Tsuen Soong (Taiwan)
John Tsiantis (Greece)
John Tse (Canada)
Betty Willett (UK)
Shoichi Watanabe (Japan)
C. Yiptong (Mauritius)

Dr. G. PERNHAUPT (Austria)

ALCOHOL AND DRUG ABUSE

The Alcohol and Drug Abuse Workshop focused on alcohol and drug abuse in Europe and North America. Participants presented papers on the treatment, consequences, and extent of alcohol and drug abuse in their respective countries. The following is a summary of the major ideas and findings contained in these papers.

A study conducted among the Pueblo tribes of New Mexico indicated that the opiate and barbiturate users felt pessimistic about their lives and future and did not care what happened to them. Heavy inhalant users did not have much self-esteem and viewed themselves as unsuccessful in the Indian way of life. The most significant finding of this study was that peer groups provided the major motivation for the young to become involved in drugs. Investigators discovered that many heavy drug users first started using inhalants under the age of eleven and under peer pressure.

During the discussion that followed this paper it was mentioned that in Europe there is especially heavy inhalant use in the Scandinavian countries. Sniffing often provides entrance to the drug scene. In Austria, inhalants are used by youngsters of low social classes and by children in schools where there is no access to other drugs. A Viennese study revealed that the earlier one starts drinking, the more likely he is to become an alcoholic. Families who tolerate their children drinking alcohol at an early age are more likely to create future alcoholics. People who start drinking between the ages of six to ten tend to become delta alcoholics (i.e., constant-level drinkers or delirium tremens-type) and to develop more somatic damage (i.e. cirrhosis of the liver).

Participants in the workshop generally agreed that identification with the drinking father is a common way of acquiring drinking habits.

The second day of the workshop dealt with various treatment approaches to alcoholism. One of the major papers on treatment pointed out that the aim of the first contact with the alcoholic is to motivate him or her to take part in a long-term treatment program, beginning with detoxification in the clinic setting. It was pointed out that it is dangerous to create the illusion that withdrawal can be achieved extramurally on the client's own terms.

In his first contact with the alcoholic, it is important to diminish feelings of shame, guilt, apprehension and distrust. The therapist should guard against becoming an extension of the alcoholic's own family, especially if the alcoholic is a child. He must not become a competitor of the family.

A second paper on treatment discussed an approach in which the early phase of treatment is based on urinary samples which the client agreed to provide. If

S. H. Fine, R. Krell, and Tsung-yi Lin (Eds.), 'Today's Priorities in Mental Health' 223–225.

the client succeeds in producing frequent clear tests, therapy is continued. If he does not continue delivering tests or if he delivers three positive tests, treatment is terminated. Client and doctor form a team as long as the client shows he is trying hard to meet the doctor's expectation.

A third paper on treatment was presented by a participant from Upper Austria, the Austrian state with the highest death rate from addiction. At this advisory and treatment centre, which maintains close contact with all other Austrian institutions handling drug problems, non-drug users are also treated but on different occasions. The main idea is that the therapist devèlops a good contact with client at the first meeting, accompanies him through detoxification at the Wagner-Jaurepp-Hospital (which has no special ward for addicts) and stays with the client in after-care as long as possible. It is of great importance in this treatment approach that there is a close personal continuity throughout all steps of detoxification and rehabilitation which may go on for several years.

In the United States there is an effort to control alcoholism and drug addiction by decriminalizing drug- and alcohol-related offences. An American paper discussed the two most important congressional laws affecting the mental health system in the United States, namely, 'The Comprehensive Mental Health Centre Act' and, 'The Alcohol Abuse and Alcoholism Act'. These Acts specifically decriminalize alcohol addiction and define it is a health problem. In response to this paper it was pointed out that in Austria the possession of drugs of any kind does not necessarily lead to imprisonment if the quantity does not exceed a certain amount which is assumed by law to be a week's ration for an addict. The Austrian person found with drugs over this amount is put under control for a year. If he is found a second time with any amount of drugs within this period, he is then sentenced.

The last day of the workshop dealt with the influence of family on drug and alcohol abuse. It was pointed out that the family is the number one factor in the development of addiction. The presenter pointed out that the absence of the father can lead to deviant behaviour. Thus, a treatment approach which emphasizes working with whole families becomes important.

The workshop concluded with a paper which compared a group of drug addicts with a representative sample from the average population. The investigators found that all risk groups had a high incidence of inadequate nurturing in childhood, separation from home, frequent change of home-caring person, and broken home situations, etc. A significant finding was that corporal punishment played an important role in the development of deviant behaviour. A cool, distant, indifferent, inconsistent, forbidding, authoritative climate was linked with later drug addiction. The paper concluded with the thought that an incomplete family situation might be better for the child than a situation of continuous conflict between parents.

In summary the general consensus of the workshop was that family and community factors have to be seriously considered to understand drug and alcohol abuse.

RESOURCE PERSONS

Jay Cutler (USA)
Dr. M. Jalali (USA)
Dr. B. Jalali (USA)
Dr. George S. Goldstein (USA)

PETER SUEDFELD, Ph.D. (Canada) and BRIAN D. THOMAS (UK)

PHYSICAL SURROUNDINGS AND ENVIRONMENTAL INFLUENCES

A number of questions, stimulated by formal presentations, were discussed during this workshop. They include: how can familial developmental tasks be reconciled with existing housing environments? Are some environments harmful to mental health – and its converse: can environmental change be used for therapeutic ends? How can behavioral science data and principles be used in architecture and design to benefit children?

Housing environments clearly affect intrafamilial transactions. However, it is difficult to devise means for testing such influences. It has been noted, for example, that pre-school children living in high-rise flats are more closely bound to their homes than children living in different conditions. The data do not show whether this phenomenon is a function of the physical environment or whether some families may use the environmental configuration to reinforce existing intrafamilial trends. Housing planning should include some mechanism for designing dwellings in a way which provides for both personal and family space. The importance of personal 'defensible' space is illustrated by the experience of North American urban renewal schemes: it has been found there that where ground was too public, it was not used. The monstrous playgrounds surrounding some housing projects probably serve to stimulate aggressive behavior and impose an increased risk of accidents.

School environments affect behavior. Large 'school factories' are undesirable for the same reasons as large 'dwelling factories'. In addition, more attention must be paid to the psychological consequences of using particular combinations of colours, materials, lighting systems, etc. Optimizing the physical aspects of therapeutic environments – particularly treatment institutions – must be balanced against the surrounding community's demand for security for itself. It has been repeatedly demonstrated that improvement in the quality of life of institutionalized patients has the effect of humanizing them and that this, in turn, can accelerate the process of making them more acceptable to the community at large. Regarding treatment settings for children, no consensus presently exists about whether mentally ill children should be treated in outpatient clinics which are separate from adult facilities; however, when they need to be hospitalized, this should be in special child psychiatric centres. Community mental health services for children must become more integrated.

Attention must be paid to a child's need to be alone. Many persons involved with education and care of children seem to feel that it is unreasonable for people to wish to be alone, that this pattern is always anti-social. However,

S. H. Fine, R. Krell, and Tsung-yi Lin (Eds.), 'Today's Priorities in Mental Health' 227–228.

in some situations a need may exist to provide children with a way to escape – at least temporarily – from environmental prisons. A school for maladjusted children in Bremen, for example, makes provisions for private space by providing curtained off alcoves into which children can retire.

The problem of improving the environment of institutionalized long-stay patients is an international one. One approach to the solution might be to provide lay monitoring of the quality of life in such institutions. If such an approach were adopted, 'check-lists' could be useful as assessment tools. The varied background and interests of lay monitors and their greater psychological accessibility to patients (and perhaps to staff members as well) are important benefits.

Although links exist between urban planners and those concerned with the physically handicapped, this is not so in mental health. The difficulty perhaps lies in the inability of those interested in the mental health field to produce quantifiable data capable of assimilation by architects and planners. This remains a high priority task for the future.

RESOURCE PERSONS

S. Kubale (Germany)
J. Piha (Finland)
S. Rudas (Austria)
J. Veroude (Holland)

GASTON HARNOIS, M.D. (Canada) and R. LACEY, (U.K.)

CHILDREN'S RIGHTS/PATIENTS' RIGHTS AND CHILD ADVOCACY

The workshop has reconstituted itself as a task force to prepare a Bill of Rights for children which will be meaningful within an international context. In order to achieve meaningfulness, it is recognized that rights must be formulated within the context of value systems.

Among the rights requiring explicit formulation, the workshop endorsed in principle the following statement of rights and responsibilities in residential treatment settings:

A DECLARATION of THE RIGHTS AND RESPONSIBILITIES OF CHILDREN IN A RESIDENTIAL CENTRE

The Centre recognizes that you have the following rights and expects each staff member to do everything in his/her power to assure you of these rights.

You are reminded that your health care is a cooperative effort between you and the staff of the Centre.

If you, or your parent, wish to contact the Patients' Rights and Ethics Committee concerning any of these rights, you may do so by personally contacting the Chairman, or by sending a letter.

It is the goal of the Centre to provide the most effective and least intrusive treatment possible in order that you and your parents, or other significant people, should have as normal a life experience as is feasible.

RIGHTS:

You have the right:

1. to be treated with respect and dignity at all times;
2. to appropriate affection and understanding;
3. to prompt medical, physical and psychological care and treatment;
4. to protection provided by qualified staff;
5. to be given all relevant information regarding your condition and treatment. If your capacity to understand is limited, your parents or guardian must be contacted and given the relevant information;
6. to some privacy;
7. to uncensored communication by letter, person or telephone;
8. to decent, safe and stimulating living conditions, nutritious food and appropriate clothing;

S. H. Fine, R. Krell, and Tsung-yi Lin (Eds.), 'Today's Priorities in Mental Health' 229–231.

9. to retain your own personal property, unless serious reasons of space, safety, value or hygiene make it impossible;
10. to the maximum of education of which you are capable in accordance with the treatment program;
11. to be exposed to moral, social, cultural and spiritual values appropriate to your age and level of functioning;
12. to play and sports activities;
13. to confidentiality of your treatment record, except when it is in your best interest to share some information with your parents or guardian;
14. to participate, or refuse to participate, in any research project. These decisions must be made with the permission of your parent or guardian;
15. to your own legal counsel;
16. to be informed of the rights of children;
17. to regular evaluation and review.

Occasionally, for therapeutic reasons, the following right may be suspended temporarily:

Number 7.

In other situations, when it is in your best interest, your parents or guardian may be consulted regarding the following rights:

Numbers 5, 13, 14.

In such situations this will be recorded in your medical chart and you will be informed of the action.

This document is a distillation of the Youth Protection Act of the Province of Quebec and is in essential agreement with the United Nations Declaration of the Rights of the Child.

RESPONSIBILITIES

In order for the greatest benefit to all people concerned, insofar as you are capable you are expected:

1. to cooperate fully and honestly with the hospital staff in your treatment and rehabilitation;
2. to abide by the rules and regulations of the institution;
3. to be responsible for your behaviour, as you are subject to all legal procedures;
4. to respect the rights and property of others;
5. to look after your physical care, i.e. bathing, grooming, dressing, etc.
6. to look after your own belongings in a reasonably orderly fashion;
7. to take advantage of the educational opportunities offered to you.

RESOURCE PERSONS

Samuel R. Fudge (USA)
Clare Marcus (USA)
Quentin Rae-Grant (Canada)
Ronald B. Rea (USA)
Rev. Douglas Wilson (Canada)

J. ERNEST RUNIONS, M.D., F.R.C.P. (C), M.R.C. (Psych.) (Canada)

RELIGION AND MENTAL HEALTH IN CHILDREN

Through a series of discussions, greatly stimulated by three informed addresses, the workshop was able to come to a consensus on aspects of religion as a force fostering mental health. The participants were quick to note and record the obvious biases in the workshop. First, nearly all represented a 'Western' cultural tradition. Second, most of the participants were coming to the workshop from an explicitly Christian tradition. The workshop could not easily explore or synthesize a broad range of views when virtually every member came from one tradition.

The discussions began with a paper entitled 'What worth the child? The child's right and health'. In summary it was stated that "Bioethical decisions affecting children are often made by considering medical/scientific, ethical and legal variables." A speaker from the U.S.A. has developed a typology of child advocacy ('Kiddy-libbers' – who hold no adult should make decisions for the child; and 'child savers' – who assert the prerogative of social institutions – especially the state – to override parents and to intervene with decisions that bind the child) which served as a useful springboard to examine the concept of children's rights. The fundamental questions raised were: who decides for the child when he cannot decide for himself? On what criteria? And what role do religious values play in these decisions? Does religion have a role at the policy level as well as at the level of individual clinical decision?

The workshop, while not able to address all of these questions, interacted with the problem of 'who decides' in regard to religious training. The members were unanimous in their opinion that the question must be answered not on an a priori ideological basis, but on the basis of a child's developing ability to make decisions. Early in a child's life parents must make a decision to teach the child religious values, attitudes and teaching if the child is to develop a religious sentiment. As the child matures, however, he must be free to test, entertain, reject, or reassemble religious ideas, without jeopardy to his relationship with his family. Religions must be taught; it must not be coerced.

While the precise content of the family's religious faith will be mediated by parents and religious workers, there are certain principles which any religious faith should show to be compatible with and contributory to the child's mental health.

Those who transmit religious ideals and teaching must have a view of humanity capable of undergirding the richness of human potential. In the opinion of workshop members a view of humanity as a noble creation, a spiritual, social and physical being, at once dependent and responsible, is essential to health; and

S. H. Fine, R. Krell, and Tsung-yi Lin (Eds.), 'Today's Priorities in Mental Health' 233–235.

neither a materialistic philosophy (or psychology) nor a pessimistic anthropology (operating from the premise that there is basically something defective about man) will foster wholeness of the person and of his relationships.

The parents' and teachers' religious view of man must also be capable of coping with the complexity of human experience: of a person's pressing biological drives and his high spiritual and moral aspirations; of his awareness of inner strength and his delicate fragility; of the richness of whole relationships and the tragedy of broken relationships; of the grace of reconciliation and the abyss of alienation.

In addition to this conceptual basis of religion, parents and teachers provide the child with a set of primary relationships. These relationships are both social and theocentric. As the workshop noted repeatedly, "We go to God with others".

In the context of relationships, guilt, fear, and anxiety can play an important role insofar as they are not neurotic (that is, arising from the person's unrecognized dissatisfaction with his own instinctual drives). The mentally healthy person will have a certain anxiety to maintain relationships (an anxiety experienced as awe in the religious dimension). Such an anxiety is free of terror, an effect that inhibits relationships.

The healthy person will also feel discomfort experienced as guilt/remorse when (s)he has been responsible for a broken relationship. This discomfort may arise from any violated relationship – whether with God or with one's fellows. Persons who do not experience guilt/remorse are seriously disabled in achieving adequate relationships (as, for example, the antisocial personality).

When personal relationships have been disrupted, the religious tradition must provide a means of reconciliation, through some form of expiation (which fully acknowledges one's responsibility in the matter) and absolution. The group reflected on the powerful healing force of a sense of forgiveness and reconciliation with God. The group was concerned not to over-individualize this experience, noting that we are social beings and must go to God in relationship with other people.

The group then turned to parental mediation of religious attitudes and precepts. In a stimulating informal address it was pointed out that religious instructors must be fully accepting of the child as a person. They demonstrate that acceptance as they communicate the tradition in terms and by means appropriate to a child's stage of perceptual, conceptual and social development.

From an early age children ask profoundly religious questions and are not satisfied with merely materialist or naturalist explanations. We are failing children – and thus putting their health in jeopardy – if we do not facilitate their approach to transcendent values and experiences through rhythmic and representative play (ages 2–5); exploring the opportunities of caring and fostering respect for life, channelling competitiveness and assisting co-operation (ages 6–12); providing opportunity for group formation around religious points of identification and for debate over religious ideas (ages 13–16); respecting religious secrets, providing trustworthy relationships in order to consolidate religious experience (ages 17–19).

It was suggested that the mentally handicapped child poses special problems to both religion and mental health. Religion must be presented to these children in concrete terms (as by the sacraments in the Christian faith), comprehensible within the child's experience. Furthermore, the child must experience the religious worker as pre-occupied with the child himself: truth is best understood through love.

To the emotionally disturbed, too, the religious content becomes valid and therapeutic as the child receives the love of catechist and the community. Religion is healthy when we go to God with others. As religion mediates love, and builds community, it becomes a positive and powerful force for mental health.

CONCLUSIONS

1. Religion facilitates mental health when it has the following characteristics:

a) a high concept of man as noble,
b) when it respects the child's stage of development and enters into the child's world, on the child's terms,
c) when it is taught in terms of the child's experience and relationships,
d) when it builds community and a network of relationships characterized by love.

2. A healthy religion builds upon personal responsibility and uses guilt, fear, etc. constructively when relationships have been broken. These emotions are used well when they become the opportunity and the means of reconciliation.

3. Parents are neglecting basic needs of children when they neglect to transmit religious values, ideals, and tradition. At the same time, the child must have, as this intellectual and emotional equipment permits, the opportunity to test and readjust his religious views without jeopardizing primary relationships.

RESOURCE PERSONS

Dr. Anne J. Davis (USA)
Rev. Dr. Euchariste Paulhus (Switzerland)
Sister Marian Delores Robinson (USA)

JOHN D. WILLIAMSON, M.B., ChB, MRCGP (U.K.)

SELF-HELP AND MUTUAL AID

Self-care, self-help and mutual aid are not the same thing (Williamson and Danaher 1978). Self-care is a huge field incorporating the maintenance of health, the prevention of disease, self-diagnosis, the negotiation of diagnosis and management of problems referred to professionals, the monitoring of disease and treatment, self-treatment, and, of course, the whole socio-political question of participation. Self-help is less pervasive than this and in its usual visage it refers to the phenomenon by which a lay person joins with others to define or meet some perceived need. The difference between self-help and mutual aid is that, whilst the latter involves a contract for reciprocal giving and taking, self-help can involve people whose problems have already been solved and so derive *less* from their involvement as a 'sufferer' and *more* from their involvement as a helper.

In these terms self-help is an essential part of the mechanism by which mutual aid groups can operate efficiently. Self-help as a term implies a greater involvement of 'healed sufferers', voluntary workers or paid, often professional, people than does mutual aid. It is, however, a distinction which is often ignored by those actually working in the field. Nevertheless this is not merely a semantic question for there is a clear difference between the approaches outlined. Even if there were no such differences, mutual aid would be the preferable term because of the peculiarly reactionary connotations of much self-help in the last century (Levin, Katz and Holtz 1976).

The mutual aid group is based on a single premise. Every member suffers a common disadvantage and is willing both to recognise and to admit this in the context of the group. The experience of suffering is critical to the dynamic of the group; the sharing of common problems builds a firm bond which is the basis of future action (Katz and Bender 1976; Robinson and Henry 1978). The involvement of non-sufferers would change the dynamic of mutual aid with the consequences of schism between helper and helped.

Self-help or mutual aid is deeply personal. It does not imply a particular set of political attitudes or social mores. When the problem is solved there is no reason for the self-helper to continue his involvement with other sufferers where he or she wants to redefine the role as a 'helper who has trod the lonely path'. Neither is there any evidence that self-helpers with one problem will have a special attitude to self-helpers suffering a different problem. Alcoholics do not help diabetics and there is no evidence that self-helping epileptics stigmatize self-helping ex-convicts – or vice-versa – any less than non-self-helping members of the community (Williamson & Danaher 1978; Katz & Bender 1976).

During one of the Plenary Sessions Professor Eisenberg was asked to comment

S. H. Fine, R. Krell, and Tsung-yi Lin (Eds.), 'Today's Priorities in Mental Health' 237–241.

on the role of mutual aid in changing social attitudes, values, behaviour. He answered to the effect that it had a substantial role which would be greater but for two reservations. First, mutual aid groups come and go rapidly without the development of a self-care ethic in the community. Second, there is a danger that people coming together in a self-help group would actually make the situation worse because society would let them take responsibility for their own condition and ignore them. The second point is the easier to argue. Experience shows that when mutual aid groups are formed they *insist* on their problem being recognized, their feelings considered, and their resource-needs met. The mental handicap lobby in America (not a benevolent politician) was responsible for the improvements in services for such people and for the change in public attitudes to handicap. The sufferers, and by this we mean the handicapped *and* their families, (Robinson and Henry 1978; Lukes 1979) did it themselves.

The development of a self-care ethic in a community depends on a large number of things. It depends on that community's reactions to the notions of self-determination or volunteerism. It depends on the level of awareness of the lay public and its educability in terms of self-care. And it depends on the alternatives available to the potential self-helper. Self-help is a political issue. The mutual aid group is a powerful tool in narrowing the gap between administrations and people, between professionals and people, and between people themselves (Danaher and Williamson 1979). Self-helpers who are successful in solving their problems through self-help or mutual aid will at least have positive attitudes to self-care. The more mutual aid groups there are, the more people will begin to develop such attitudes. If groups can be developed for people with problems at that most formative stage, adolescence, then increasing numbers of adults with positive ideas will be generated (Williamson 1979). If a self-help or mutual aid group can be introduced into a network of such groups it is possible that the lack of interest in one set of self-helpers in the problems, or interests, of other self-helpers will be countered (Ariel 1978).

Certainly it is clear that the mutual aid movement can help to change people's attitudes of particular problems. Not only can reactions to stigmatizing conditions be raised (Khantavichian 1979), but also public reaction to stigmatizing behaviours (like masturbation) can be changed by using these as therapeutic weapons in attacking a non-stigmatized problem through self-help (Czerwenka-Wenkstetten 1979). Alcoholics Anonymous has done more to change public attitudes to alcoholism than any professional group (Kropotkin 1955).

A significant problem for further discussion is the relationship of self-helpers to outsiders, particularly professionals, who are introduced into the group. There is an obvious danger that as an outsider's contribution increases there is a consequent diminishing in that of the self-helpers, first the 'ordinary' membership and then the informal power structure of the group (Williamson 1979). But professionals and others *can*, and need to, avoid taking groups over (Williamson 1979) and they can act in such a way as to promote the self-care ethic. This will require them to avoid personalizing the orientation of the group with regard to professional intervention and it will require them to be prepared to stand as consultants to the group rather than participants (Schmidt 1979). It is important to stress that no outsider should personalize his or her involvement by taking on a therapeutic role in relation to one or more of the self-helpers. To fall into this trap is to convert the mutual aid group into an ad hoc therapy group; the result being that it will first professionalize, then beaurocratize into a living fossil (Katz 1979).

A second major problem relates to the question of how planners and service providers can encourage the establishment of mutual aid groups in their communities. A number of approaches suggest themselves. First, the professions can engage in mutual aid to answer their own problem. A problem of uncertainty or insecurity in performing one's work is as valid a disadvantage as blindness; both are amenable to self-help (Williamson and Danaher 1978; Levin, Katz and Holst 1976). Second, the professionals can encourage the community to see its own problems in self-help terms, either by going out into the community (Danaher and Williamson 1979; Gochman and Gochman 1979) or by making themselves available so that members of the community could come to them (Ariel 1978; Richards, Williamson and Windass 1979). Third, they can tap the resources of national voluntary agencies to see if these might identify problems amenable to self-help which could be highlighted in their normal educational or social gatherings (National Childbirth Trust (UK) 1979).

There must be many other valid initiatives that caring professionals can make to encourage mutual aid but these have yet to be described. However, there is one situation in which self-help is particularly viable as a complement and an alternative to professional care. In war or other armed conflicts normal social and professional standards are suspended (Minkowski 1979). Self-help is a matter of survival. The ratio of stress to available supportive structures is optimal (Halpern 1979; Burns 1979). This illustrates one major, general principle; that in planning communities the architects and designers should avoid the temptation to manipulate people. If the physical environment is capable of manipulation by the people living in it, it is much more likely that they will react positively to the challenge of self-determination however that is expressed (Danaher and Williamson 1979). The question is how to motivate people to be self-determined.

The real challenge for those interested in mental health is this motivation. Many of the issues identified as contributing to the community's mental health require a massive shift in social attitudes, values and behaviours. The typical response is to throw up hands in despair and build yet another social institution to educate or serve. But we do not need more institutions. They inhibit people's self-determinism and they undermine people's self-sufficiency. Talking about social change does not make it happen; but talking can help to generate an environment in which change is possible. Social change is effected by those who believe it is needed. If the people want to change and the environment is right, then change will take place. The professional and the enlightened, caring laypersons have major roles in encouraging their fellow human-beings to express *their own* needs and to advise *their own* strategies for meeting these. Self-care, self-help and mutual aid are not the complete answer to our most pressing social problems, but they have a potential which it would be foolish to ignore.

RESOURCE PERSONS

J. Burns (UK)
G. Czerwenka-Wenkstetten (Austria)
K. Danaher (UK)
E. R. Gochman (USA)
S. Gochman (Puerto Rico)
E. Halpern (Israel)
S. Khantavichian (Thailand)
M. Lukes (Australia)
A. Minkowski (France)
National Childbirth Trust (UK)
R. Schmidt (UK)

REFERENCES

Ariel
1978 Factsheet describing the aims and objectives of a Community Self-Help Resource Centre, UK: Barnstey.

Burns, J.
1979 Caring and Sharing. Contribution to the workshop.

Czerwenka-Wenkstetten, G.
1979 Autoerotic Training for People with Psychosomatic Problems. Contribution to the workshop.

Danaher, K. and Williamson, J. D.
1979 New Town Blues: Planning and Mutual Aid. Contribution to the workshop.

Gochman, E. R. and Gochman, S.
1979 Explorations in Community Psychology in the Development of Communities. Contribution to the workshop.

Helpern, E.
1979 Stress in War Orphans, (summary title). Contribution to the workshop.

Katz, A. H. and Bender, E. I.
1976 The Strength in Us: Self Help Groups in the Modern World. New Viewpoints, New York and London: Franklin-Watts.

Katz, A. H.
1979 Personal Communication, Article in Press.

Khantavichian, S.
1979 Contribution to the workshop.

Kropotkin, P.
1955 Mutual Aid: A Factor of Evolution. Boston: Extending Horizons Books.

Levin, L., Katz, A. H. and Holst, E.
1976 Self Care: Lay Initiatives in Health. New York: Prodist.

Lukes, M.
1979 An Association for Relatives and Families of the Mentally Ill. Contribution to the workshop.

Minkowski, A.
1979 Experiences of self-help in conflict. Contribution to the workshop.

National Childbirth Trust (UK)
1979 Motherhood, Fatherhood, Growing into Parenthood. Contribution to the workshop.

Richards, J., Williamson, J. D. and Windass, S.
1979 Neighbourhood Health. Osford and London: Anglo-German Foundation for Alternatives.

Robinson, D. and Henry, S.
1978 Self Help in Health. London: Martin Robertson.
Schmidt, R.
1979 Hearing the Child in the Adult. Contribution to the workshop.
Williamson, J. D. and Danaher, K.
1978 Self Care in Health. London: Croom-Helm.
Williamson, J. D.
1979 Adolescent Medicine and Mutual Aid. Contribution to the workshop.
Williamson, J. D.
1979 The Lay/Professional Interface in Mutual Aid, in "Self Help and Mutual Aid in the Health and Social Services" (ed. S. Hatch). London: Volunteer Centre (NCCS).

INDEX OF NAMES

INDEX OF SUBJECTS

GPSR Compliance

The European Union's (EU) General Product Safety Regulation (GPSR) is a set of rules that requires consumer products to be safe and our obligations to ensure this.

If you have any concerns about our products, you can contact us on ProductSafety@springernature.com

In case Publisher is established outside the EU, the EU authorized representative is:

Springer Nature Customer Service Center GmbH
Europaplatz 3
69115 Heidelberg, Germany

Batch number: 10607222

Printed by Printforce, the Netherlands